CLINICAL MICROBIOLOGY REVIEW

Second Edition   Peter Q. Warinner, MD

Self-assessment review questions visit: **www.wysteria.com**

D1404573

COVER ART: *Winlochan At Midnight* by Elizabeth H. Fleitas

WYSTERIA
Long Island, New York

Library of Congress Cataloging-in-Publication Data

Warinner, Peter Q.
    Clinical microbiology review / Peter Q. Warinner. -- 2nd ed.
       p. cm.
    Includes index.
    ISBN 0-9651162-1-2 (alk. paper)
    1. Medical microbiology--Outlines, syllabi, etc. I. Title.
    [DNLM: 1. Microbiology--handbooks. 2. Microbiology--outlines.
3. Communicable Diseases--handbooks. 4. Communicable Diseases-
-outlines.   QW 39 W277c 1998]
QR46.W28   1998
616'.01--dc21
DNLM/DLC
for Library of Congress   97-46073
                                    CIP

Printed in the U.S.A.

ACKNOWLEDGMENTS:

For their inspiration, advice and support:

    Doris J. Bucher, Ph.D.
    Associate Professor of Microbiology & Immunology
    New York Medical College, NY

    Soldano Ferrone, M.D., Ph.D.
    Chairman, Department of Microbiology & Immunology
    New York Medical College, NY

    Gary P. Wormser, M.D.
    Professor of Medicine and Pharmacology
    Chief, Division of Infectious Disease
    New York Medical College
    Westchester County Medical Center, NY

For use of their microorganism specimen collections:

    Maria E. Aguero-Rosenfeld, M.D.
    Associate Professor of Pathology
    New York Medical College
    Associate Director of Clinical Pathology
    Westchester County Medical Center, NY

    Dr. Joseph S. Tatz
    Assistant Clinical Professor
    Department of Pathology
    Westchester County Medical Center, NY

This book is dedicated to the hope that medical research will find the way to cure or prevent HIV infection.

A portion of the proceeds from the sale of this book will be donated to HIV research.

HOW TO USE THIS BOOK

There is an overwhelming amount of confusing and somewhat disorganized information to be learned in the study of medical microbiology. This review book will provide clarity, organization and simplicity.

1. Wherever possible, organisms are categorized according to the diseases they cause or according to certain common distinguishing features.
2. With only one exception, each pathogen is presented entirely on one page or less so that the reader can focus without the need to turn pages.
3. Information is brief, to the point, and corresponds well to standardized exam questions.
4. High-yield information is highlighted in **bold type** for easy scanning.
5. Cross references are presented at the end of each section; and a general cross reference is presented at the end of the last section.
6. Every-other page is left blank so that notes can be added right next to the appropriate pathogen or cross reference area.
7. It is helpful to consolidate all extraneous notes into this one book, as a journal, to provide for a rapid comprehensive review whenever needed.

8. The **color coding** is intended as a memory aid. The code is as follows:
   (**Note**: Other patterns will become recognizable while using the book.)

Gram Positive Bacteria	Blue
Gram Negative Bacteria	Red
Acid Fast Bacteria	Purple
Spirochetes	Green
Chlamydia and Mycoplasma	Black
DNA Viruses	Blue
RNA Viruses	Red
Prions	Black
Fungi	Green
Protozoa Parasites	Red
Helminth Parasites	Blue

NOTE: All corrections and suggestions should be sent c/o Wysteria Publishing, P.O. Box 470, Freeport, NY 11520. Via Email: **wysteria@wysteria.com**

TABLE OF CONTENTS:

Chapter 1

BASIC TERMINOLOGY REVIEW

CELL WALL: contains peptidoglycan:

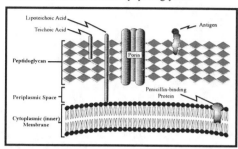

GRAM POSITIVE

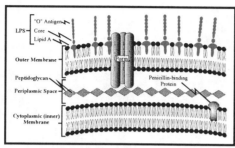

GRAM NEGATIVE

OXYGEN REQUIREMENTS for the pathogen:

Obligate Aerobic: Requires presence of oxygen.
Aerobic (facultative):   Prefers the presence of oxygen, but tolerates absence.
Microaerophilic: Grows only in less than atmospheric level of oxygen.
Anaerobic (facultative):   Prefers absence of oxygen, but tolerates presence.
Obligate Anaerobic: Requires absence of oxygen.

GROWTH ENVIRONMENT for the pathogen within the host:

Extracellular: Prefer to exist outside of host cells, may adhere to, or move between, host cells.
Intracellular: Prefer to exist inside of host cells, but can survive outside.
Obligate Intracellular: Requires intracellular environment for survival, cannot survive outside.

Invasive: this term is used to indicate the ability of a pathogen to penetrate the membranes and tissues of the host's body. For example, a non-invasive pathogen will remain in the intestinal lumen, but an invasive pathogen will penetrate the intestinal epithelium. Invasive pathogens may be extracellular (moving between host cells) or intracellular (moving through host cells).

FEATURES

Microscopic characteristics:
     Morphology: coccus (spheres), coccobacillus, bacillus (rods), spirochete, "club," "boxcar," etc.
     Grouping: pairs, chains, clusters, filamentous, "coffee bean pairs," "Chinese-character clumps," etc.
Culture characteristics:
     Media: blood agar, chocolate agar, special additives, etc.
     Conditions: aerobic, anaerobic.
     Cell culture (tissue culture): necessary for obligate intracellular pathogens.
     Colony characteristics: color, speed of growth, size, shape, "swarming", etc.

MOTILITY

1. Non-motile
2. Flagellated Motility:

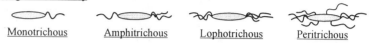

Monotrichous   Amphitrichous   Lophotrichous   Peritrichous

3. Other Motility: tumble, corkscrew, darting, twitching, rotating, etc.

CAPSULES: extra coat that tightly surrounds bacteria to enhance survival (promotes adhesion, resists antibiotics, resists phagocytosis). Composition varies: polysaccharide, polypeptide, lipid, protein, etc.

GLYCOCALYX: also known as "slime layer" or exopolysaccharide: material that loosely coats bacteria to enhance survival (promotes adhesion, resists antibiotics, resists phagocytosis).

SPORES: special dormancy state that enhances long-term survival in extremely harsh conditions. Special conditions are required for germination back to normal metabolic state.

TOXINS (see treatment section below for explanation of toxoid and antitoxin):

Exotoxin: This is a toxic substance produced and released by the pathogen into the surrounding environment.
     e.g. Enterotoxin: a type of exotoxin that has its effect on the GI tract.
     e.g. Neurotoxin: a type of exotoxin that has its effect on the nervous system.
Food Poisoning in most cases, is caused by an exotoxin that is "pre-formed" by the pathogen in the food before the host eats the food. It is the toxin, not the pathogen that causes the illness.
Endotoxin: This is a species-specific lipopolysaccharide (LPS) molecule that is built into the outer membrane of gram negative bacteria. Endotoxin is released upon disruption of membrane. Each LPS is made up of a polysaccharide "O" unit for antigenic variation, and a phospholipid "Lipid A" unit for toxicity.

BACTERIAL GENETICS

Plasmid: circular, self-replicating, extra-chromosomal bacterial DNA which caries genes for antibiotic resistance (R-plasmid), genes for conjugation (F-plasmid), genes for toxins, and other non-essential products.

Conjugation: "males" possess "F-factor" on plasmid; male gives copy of plasmid to "female" via male sex pilus. "Female" gains possession of plasmid genetic material including the "F-factor;" thereby becomes "male."

High-Frequency Recombination (Hfr) conjugation: the "F-factor" is coded on the male chromosome, not plasmid. During conjugation, female gains possession of some male chromosomal genetic material along with F-factor.

Bacteriophage ("phage"): a virus that infects bacteria.

Lytic Transduction: phage-infected bacteria ruptures; the phage picks up some bacterial DNA; the phage infects another bacteria and inserts the new DNA.

Lysogenic Transduction: phage-infected bacteria gets pieces of it's DNA excised; those pieces get incorporated into the phage as the phage re-assembles and exits (without lysis of host bacteria); the same phage then infects a new bacteria and inserts DNA from the first bacteria.

SOURCE AND DEFINITION OF INFECTION

Pathogen: a disease-causing organism.

Host: a person who temporarily harbors organisms.

Reservoir: the place where a pathogen lives naturally: the soil, an animal's blood stream, a human colon, etc.

Colony: when organisms temporarily survive in a place outside their normal habitat, but cause no disease.

    Colonization may occur on inanimate objects (fomites), or within a human host.

Commensal organism: ("Normal Flora"): an organism that lives harmlessly at a specific site within a human host.

    Note: commensal organisms may become pathogens when they move to a different location within the host.

Carrier: a person who unnaturally harbors a pathogen, for a long period of time, but exhibits no symptoms of the disease. The carrier may be capable of transmitting the pathogen (and the disease) to another person.

Infection: the condition whereby colonization within a human host causes disease.

Transmissible: the ability of an infection to spread from one person to another.

Contagious: the concept that a disease can be transmissible.

Communicable: the concept that a disease can be transmissible.

ROUTES OF TRANSMISSION

Iatrogenic: caused by health-care professional as result of some treatment or procedure.

Nosocomial: acquired within the hospital environment.

Community acquired: acquired outside the hospital environment.

Horizontal: transmission of infection from person to person:

    Direct Contact; Respiratory droplets; Fecal-Oral route; Sexually Transmitted Disease (STD); etc.

Vertical: infected mother transmits to her unborn/newborn child.

    1. In-utero:

        Across placenta.

        Ascending to uterus from vagina.

    2. At birth:

        Passage through vagina.

    3. After birth:

        Breast-feeding.

Vector-borne: pathogens are introduced into the host by intervention of some insect. The insect is the vector. The reservoir for vector-borne pathogens is usually some animal. The human is the host.

Zoonotic: zoonotic pathogens have animals as their reservoirs, infection is spread to human hosts by direct contact with the animals; by animal bites or scratches; by drinking water that was exposed to animal urine or feces; or by ingestion of food products made from the animals; In some cases, once a human is infected, some horizontal or vertical transmission may occur.

Exogenous: infection comes from source outside the host's body.

Endogenous: infection comes from source within the host's own body.

    Direct Extension.

    Hematological spread.

    Lymphangytic spread.

    Ascending (e.g. Via urethra to Kidney, etc.).

    Aspiration into respiratory tract from regurgitation or from lack of cough response.

    Auto-inoculation: infection transferred from one place on the host's body to another place on the host's body, usually carried on hand after touching the infected site; or via fecal-urinary route due to poor hygiene; etc.

TYPES OF INFECTION

Incubation of infection: the time period between initial contact with the pathogen and the onset of symptoms.

Local infection: infection confined to a specific site or organ.

Systemic infection: infection spreading throughout the body via bloodstream or lymphatics.

Disseminated infection: same as systemic.

Acute infection: severe symptoms manifest over a short period of time (days, weeks).

Subacute infection: mild symptoms manifest over a period of months.

Chronic infection: symptoms manifest over a long period of time (month, years).

Persistent infection: an active infection which continues in spite of typically effective treatment.

Recrudescent: symptoms relent for a brief period (days, weeks) then return. The infection is continuous.

Relapse: symptoms relent for a long period (weeks, months) then return. The infection is continuous even though it appeared to go away.

Latency: when the infecting pathogen goes into a period of dormancy within the host, symptoms relent for very long periods (months, years, decades). The infection is continuous. This is the period before reactivation.

Reactivation: the infecting pathogen remains dormant somewhere within the host for a long period of time (months, years, decades) then becomes active again to cause symptoms.

Reinfection: a new infection that occurs after a previous infection with the same pathogen had fully resolved. Or: new infection of an organ after previous infection of same organ had fully resolved, regardless of pathogen.

Recurrent: same as reinfection.

Mixed: infection with many types of pathogens, often said of a combination of anaerobes and aerobes.

Co-infection: the requirement that two pathogens be present within a host at the same time in order to produce disease (the one on its own will cause no disease).

Superinfection: the condition whereby a new pathogen is introduced at the same site where there is a pre-existing infection caused by a different pathogen. The first pathogen may alter the host in such a way as to permit the second one to thrive. The second pathogen may cause symptoms that differ from the pre-existing infection.

Opportunistic: the condition whereby a relatively non-virulent pathogen manages to cause disease in a host who is immunocompromised. The same pathogen would cause no disease in an immunocompetent host.

Endemic: status within a particular geographic area or particular subset population whereby a pathogen infects a fixed percentage of persons. As one person heals, another becomes infected; percentage of infected remains approximately constant.

Epidemic (a.k.a. "outbreak"): status within a particular geographic area or particular subset population whereby a pathogen infects an increasing percentage of persons over a relatively short period of time.

Pandemic: an epidemic that spreads across continents.

-emia: (bacteremia, viremia, spirochetemia, fungemia, parasitemia, etc.): presence of organisms in the host's bloodstream with no systemic symptoms.

Sepsis (a.k.a. septicemia): presence of pathogens and/or their toxins in the host bloodstream with concurrent constitutional symptoms (fever, tachycardia, tachypnea, increased white cell count).

Pyogenic: infection by pathogen that causes pus (inflammatory response).

Pyrogenic: infection by pathogen that causes fever.

Suppurative: infection by pathogen that causes pus (inflammatory response).

Post-infectious, non-suppurative sequelae: a type of affliction that arises within a host after an infection has fully resolved and after the infecting pathogen has been fully cleared from the host's body. This type of affliction may be caused by a delayed and abnormal autoimmune response to the previously infecting pathogen.

TYPES OF HOSTS

<u>Immunocompetent</u>: person with normal functioning immune system.

<u>Immunocompromised</u>: broad term which encompasses the following terms:

<u>Immunodeficient</u>: person whose immune system is abnormal, due to endogenous process.

<u>Immunoincompetent</u>: same as Immunodeficient.

<u>Immunosupressed</u>: person whose immune system is adversely affected by medications, radiation, or some other exogenous process.

<u>Immunodepressed</u>: same as immunosupressed.

Examples of immunocompromised states:

1. AIDS (destroys T-cells).
2. Chemotherapy which disrupts hematopoiesis (suppresses bone marrow).
3. Radiation which disrupts hematopoiesis (suppresses bone marrow).
4. Long term immunosuppressive medication given due to organ transplantation.
5. Congenital immunodeficiency.
6. Splenectomy (allows infection by encapsulated organisms).
7. Trauma (disrupted anatomic barriers).
Etc.

VIRULENCE FACTORS (Features to enhance the pathogen's survival and promote invasion of the host):

Toxins
Capsules
Enzymes
Motility
Rapid proliferation
Drug resistance
Attachment ability
Antigen variation.
Etc.

TREATMENTS

<u>Active</u>: Antimicrobial medications.

<u>Supportive</u>: respiratory ventilation; fluid resuscitation, etc.

<u>Preventive</u>:

1. <u>Acquired Immunity</u>: form of active immunity when previous infection confers long lasting immunity.
2. <u>Active Immunization</u>: form of active immunity that takes weeks or months to develop.
    Vaccines:
        <u>Live-attenuated</u>: living but inactive pathogens are injected into the host to stimulate host immunity but cause no disease.
        <u>Dead</u>: parts of dead pathogens are injected into the host to stimulate host immunity.
        <u>Toxoid</u>: inactivated exotoxin is injected into host to stimulate host immunity against the toxin. The host will form antibodies to the toxin ("antitoxin").
3. <u>Passive Immunization</u>:form of passive immunity that is immediately effective
    <u>Donor Antibody Transfer</u>: pre-formed pathogen-specific antibody is removed from an immune donor and intravenously injected into a non-immune host after the host has been exposed to a deadly pathogen.
    <u>Antitoxins</u>. pre-formed exotoxin-specific antibody is removed from an immune donor (human or animal) and intravenously injected into a non-immune host after the host has been exposed to a deadly exotoxin.
4. <u>Herd Immunity</u>: the concept that vaccination of most members of a community will decrease the likelihood that a non-immune person will come in contact with an infecting pathogen.
5. <u>Destruction of pathogen's Vector or Reservoir</u>: e.g. Fight *Yersinia pestis* by using insecticides to kill the flea vectors, and by using rat poison to kill the rat reservoir.
6. <u>Destruction of pathogen's habitat</u>: e.g. Fight *Staphylococcus aureus* by washing hospital surfaces with alcohol.

HOST DEFENSE

<u>Anatomic/Natural</u>: skin, mucous membranes, secretions, etc.

<u>Humoral</u>: Immune globulin antibodies IgM, IgG, IgA

<u>Titer</u>: to measure a host's level of a specific antibody, a sample of the host's serum is removed then put through a series of dilutions; the point of greatest dilution which still reacts in an antibody-antigen reaction is called the "titer." The greater the dilution = "higher titer" = higher antibody level.

<u>Cell-mediated</u>: CD4 T-cells, CD8 T-cells.

<u>Opsonization</u> by IgG; C3b; IgM+C3b; or IgG+C3b.

<u>Phagocytosis</u> by PMNs or MACROs.

<u>Cytokines</u> released.

<u>Compliment</u>:

<u>Classic pathway</u> (antibody dependent)

<u>Alternative path</u> (antibody independent)

<u>C5a chemotactic signal</u>: attracts phagocytes.

<u>Previous infection</u> may or may not result in:

<u>Type-specific-immunity</u>: host becomes immune to the specific strain of that species

<u>Cross-immunity</u>: host becomes immune to that specific species as well as to other similar species.

<u>Auto-Immune reaction</u>: host antibodies attack "self" tissue believing that it is an invading pathogen.

DIAGNOSTIC TESTS

A. Obtain Specimens:
> Throat swabs
> Sputum smear
> Blood smear or culture
> CSF slide or culture
> Tissue biopsy
> Urine sample slide or culture
> Urethral discharge slide or culture
> Vaginal discharge slide or culture
> Stool sample slide or culture
> Joint tap synovial fluid slide or culture
> Any Body Cavity fluid slide or culture

Contamination of Specimen: organisms, from the environment, that grow in culture along with the infecting pathogen.

B. DIRECT DETECTION OF PATHOGENS WITHIN A SPECIMEN:
Staining Methods:
1. Histological Slides:
Gram Stain for bacteria.
> Organisms are G-POS (blue/purple) or G-NEG (red).
Giemsa Stain: for miscellaneous blood smears and for protozoa.
> Organisms are pink/purple.
Silver Stain (GBS or Grocott-Gomori methenamine-silver nitrate) for fungi in tissue:
> Fungi are brown against green background.
Wright Stain: for malarial parasites.
Ziehl-Neelsen and Kinyoun ("acid-fast") for Mycobacteria.
> "Modified" for Nocardia and Cryptosporidium.
> Organisms are purple against blue background.
Etc.
2. Immunoassay Methods:
These methods depend on antigen-antibody reactions. Typically, the infecting pathogen has a specific antigen that an antibody can target. Commercially available antibody is designed in such a way that it carries a "label," or in such a way that it can be "labeled" at a later time. The label is what indicates that a positive reaction has occurred.
> Radioactive Immunoassay (RIA): the "label" is a radioactive molecule.
> Immunofluorescence Assay (IFA): the "label" is a fluorescent molecule.
> Enzyme-Linked Immunoassay (EIA) e.g. ELISA: the "label" is an enzyme which can react in a colorometric reaction.
> LA (Latex Particle Agglutination): the "label" is a large latex particle coated with antibody so that organisms which express the specific antigen will all attach to the particle.
3. DNA Probe with PCR amplification:
A "probe" DNA sequence is artificially constructed to exactly compliment the infecting pathogen's DNA. This artificial DNA probe carries a "label." The infecting pathogen's DNA is seperated into single strands, then amplified by PCR. The artificial DNA probe is introduced; complimentary matching strands will bind with the probe ("Hybridize"). The label is what indicates a positive match.

C. INDIRECT DETECTION OF PATHOGENS IN A HOST:
1. Serological Methods:
When the host becomes infected, specific antibodies are produced. In general, the IgM Titer begins to rise within 1-2 weeks and peaks after about 4 weeks then drops to a low level. In general, the IgG Titer begins to rise within 4 weeks and peaks after about 6 weeks, but persists for many years. Serologic tests are used to detect a 4 fold rise in antibody titers within two blood samples drawn about 2 weeks apart near the beginning of an infection.

2. Culture Techniques:
The tissue or body fluid specimen is introduced to special nutritive medias and incubated under special conditions. In time, bacterial colonies may grow. The bacteria from these colonies are used to conduct a series of laboratory tests for exact identification of the infecting pathogen.
Cell Culture (also called Tissue Culture) techniques are similar to regular culture techniques except that the infecting pathogens require the presence of living cells or tissue in order to survive in culture.

D. LABORATORY TESTS:
Infecting pathogens that are grown in culture can be put through numerous tests for exact identification. Tests such as: Catalase, Oxidase, Urease, Lactase, Indole, Methyl Red, Hemolysis, CAMP test, Bile-solubility, Lancefield Group, antibiotic susceptibility, etc., etc. are sometimes necessary.

Chapter 2

GRAM POSITIVE COCCI

Staphylococcus aureus
Skin infections
Food poisong
Toxic shock syndrome
Osteomyelitis
Infective arthritis
Acute endocarditis
Pneumonia
Sepsis
Parotitis

Staphylococcus epidermidis
Bacteremia
Sub-acute endocarditis
Neonatal bacteremia

Staphylococcus saprophyticus
UTI

Streptococcus Group A   Skin infections
Necrotizing fasciitis
Pharyngitis
Scarlet fever
Acute glomerular nephritis
Acute rheumatic fever

Streptococcus Group B   Neonate meningitis
Neonate pneumonia
Post-partum endometritis

Streptococcus pneumoniae
Lobar pneumonia
Meningitis
Sinusitis
Otitis media

Streptococcus Group D
(*S. bovis* and others)   Bacteremia
Sub acute endocarditis
Colon cancer

Streptococcus Viridans Group
(*S. mutans* and others)   Sub-acute endocarditis
Dental caries

Enterococcus spp
(*E. faecalis* and others)
UTI
Bacteremia
Sub-acute endocarditis

Peptostreptococcus spp (Anaerobic)
(see Commensal Anaeroic Bacteria chapter)

Staphylococcus aureus

GRAM STAIN:
POS

AEROBIC

EXTRACELLULAR

FEATURES:
- Cocci : **clusters**.
- Colonies: white/yellow, round on blood-agar.

MOTILITY:
None

CAPSULE & GLYCOCALYX:
None

EXOTOXINS:
- **Hemolysins:** (disrupt blood cells)
  - **Alpha toxin:** causes septic shock and dermonecrosis, and causes some lysis of RBC's
  - **Beta toxin:** sphingomyelinase activity. Causes lysis of RBC's in the cold after warm incubation. Basis of CAMP Test.
  - **Delta toxin:** Leukocidin activity.
  - **Gamma toxin:** causes tissue necrosis
- **Panton-Valentine Leukocidin:** (aka P-V Leukocidin)
  - Disrupts PMNs and Macros.
  - Causes influx of Ca^{++} then degranulation and lysis.
- **Enterotoxins:** (disrupts intestinal mucosa, causes emesis and diarrhea)
  - **Toxin A:** preformed in food, causes food poisoning.
  - **Toxin F:** similar to Toxic Shock Syndrome Toxin.
- **Toxic Shock Syndrome Toxin:** Superantigen.
  - Causes the release of Il-2 from CD4+ T-cells and IL-1 from Macrophages.
- **Exfoliatin:** (produced by "Phage Group II" strains) Epidermolytic.
  - Causes intraepidermal separation at stratum granulosum.

CLINICAL:
- **Skin Infections:**
  - **Furuncles, Boils, Carbuncles.**
  - **Scalded Skin Syndrome** in young children (Ritter's disease).
  - **Burn** and **wound** infections.
- **Food Poisoning:** patient ingests **Enterotoxin A** in food, not the bacteria.
  - Symptoms: nausea and vomiting.
- **Toxic Shock Syndrome:** mostly in women during use of **tampons**.
- **Osteomyelitis:** (*S. aureus* is # 1 causative organism)
  - In metaphysis of children, epiphysis of adults.
  - From trauma or hematogenous spread.
- **Infective Arthritis:** (*S. aureus* is # 1 causative organism in adults)
- **Acute Endocarditis:** (*S. aureus* is # 1 causative organism)
  - Infects normal, abnormal and prosthetic heart valves.
- **Post Viral Lobar Pneumonia:** especially following Influenza virus.
- **Bacteremia and Sepsis:** (*S. aureus* is # 1 causative organism)
  - Community acquired.
- **Parotitis:**
  - Infection of the parotid gland and duct of Stensen.

SOURCE & TRANSMISSION:
- Colonizes **human nose**, sometimes skin; may also survive on contaminated fomites, and on contaminated food.
- Horizontal transmission occurs via **human contact**, **sneezes**, and contact with the contaminated environment.
- **Nosocomial** transmission is very common.

VIRULENCE FACTORS:
- **Exotoxins**
- **β-Lactamase** coded on Plasmid: for Penicillin resistance.
- **Mutant Penicillin-Binding-Proteins:** for Methicillin resistance.
- **Coagulase** (free or bound): catalyzes the formation of thrombin which catalyzes the formation of fibrin which coats the bacteria.
- **Protein A:** binds Fc portion of IgG to block complement binding and block opsonization.
- Other Enzymes: Lipase, Protease, Hyaluronidase, nuclease, fibrinolysin.

TREATMENT:
- **Nafcillin** or other penicillinase-resistant penicillin.
- **Vancomycin**
- **Cephalosporins**, 1st Generation.
- Topical **Bacitracin** Prophylaxis

VACCINE & TOXOID:
None

HOST DEFENSE & IMMUNITY:
- Opsonization by **IgG, C3b,** or **IgM+C3b** then phagocytosis by **PMNs**.
- CD4+ T-cells release **cytokines**.
- No immunity gained by infection.

LAB TESTS:
- **Catalase:** Pos
- **Coagulase:** Pos
- **DNase:** Pos
- **Mannitol:** Pos
- Hemolysis: Beta
- **6.5%NaCl:** Growth

Staphylococcus epidermidis

GRAM STAIN:
POS

AEROBIC

EXTRACELLULAR

FEATURES:
- Cocci: Clusters.
- Colonies: White, round on Blood-Agar.

MOTILITY:
None

CAPSULE & GLYCOCALYX:
- **Glycocalyx only:** Exopolysaccharide

EXOTOXINS:
None

CLINICAL:
- **Bacteremia and Sepsis:**
  - **Nosocomial/ Iatrogenic:** catheters, IV lines, feeding tubes, prosthetics (heart valves, hip joints, pace makers, etc.), CSF shunts.
  - **Drug Abusers:** from IV injections.
  - In **immunocompromised** and neutropenic patients.
- **Subacute Endocarditis:**
  - Results from bacteremia.
  - Infects only abnormal valves or prosthetic valves.
- **Neonatal Bacteremia:**
  - Nosocomial, especially in neonatal ICUs.

SOURCE & TRANSMISSION:
- **Normal flora** of skin and mucus membranes.
- Spreads to blood following skin trauma.

VIRULENCE FACTORS:
- **Glycocalyx:** the exopolysaccharide **"slime"** enables adhesion, resistance to phagocytosis, and resistance to antibiotics.
- **β-Lactamase** coded on plasmid: for Penicillin resistance.
- **Mutant Penicillin-Binding-Proteins:** for Methicillin resistance.

TREATMENT:
- **Vancomycin**

VACCINE & TOXOID:
None

HOST DEFENSE & IMMUNITY:
- Opsonization by IgG, C3b, or IgM+C3b then phagocytosis by PMNs.
- CD4+ T-cells release cytokines.
- No immunity gained by infection.

LAB TESTS:
- **Catalase:** Pos
- Coagulase: Neg
- DNase: Neg
- Mannitol: Neg
- Hemolysis: None
- **Novobiocin** **Susceptible**

Staphylococcus saprophyticus

GRAM STAIN:
POS

AEROBIC

EXTRACELLULAR

FEATURES:
- Cocci : Clusters.
- Colonies: White/yellow, round on Blood-Agar.

MOTILITY:
None

CAPSULE & GLYCOCALYX:
None

EXOTOXINS:

None

CLINICAL:
- UTI:
  - Upper (**pyelonephritis**) and lower (**cystitis**) urinary tract infections.
  - Most cases show **pyuria**
  - Mostly in healthy, young, **sexually-active women.**

SOURCE & TRANSMISSION:
- **Normal flora** of genitourinary skin
- Spreads to urinary tract due to poor hygiene, especially related to sexual activity.

VIRULENCE FACTORS:
- Multiple drug resistance.
- Hemagglutinin proteins and surface proteins may mediate attachment to urinary tract epithelial cells.
- Urease may mediate pathogenesis.

TREATMENT:
- **Trimethoprim-Sulfamethoxazole**

VACCINE & TOXOID:

None

HOST DEFENSE & IMMUNITY:
- Opsonization by IgG, C3b, or IgM+C3b then phagocytosis by PMNs.
- CD4+ T-cells release cytokines.
- No immunity gained by infection.

LAB TESTS:
- **Catalase:** **Pos**
- Coagulase: Neg
- DNase: Neg
- Mannitol: Neg
- Hemolysis: None
- **Novobiocin** **Resistant**

Streptococcus Group A (pyogenes)

GRAM STAIN:
POS

AEROBIC

EXTRACELLULAR

FEATURES:
- Cocci : Chains.
- Colonies: small, gray-white on Blood-Agar.

MOTILITY:
None

CAPSULE & GLYCOCALYX:
- **Capsule:**
  Hyaluronic acid

EXOTOXINS:
- **Hemolysins:** (disrupt blood cells)
  - **Streptolysin O:** causes beta hemolysis.
    Inactivated by oxidation.
    Causes host immune system to produce antibody "ASO."
  - **Streptolysin S:** causes beta hemolysis on blood-agar plates.
    Resists inactivation by oxidation.
    Non-antigenic, but may have leukocidin activity.
- **Erythrogenic Toxin:** produces an erythematous reaction.
  - Causes the **Rash of Scarlet Fever**.
  - Coded on viral DNA which gets integrated into the bacteria by **lysogeny** (the process whereby a temperate bacteriophage infects a bacterium).

CLINICAL:
- **Skin Infections:**
  - **Impetigo** (Streptococcal Pyoderma): purulent with crusting
  - **Cellulitis:** (#1 causative organism) **GAS** cellulitis infects wounds such as burns , trauma, and IV drug abuser injection sites.
  - **Erysipelas:** mostly of the face, **"slapped cheek"** rash.
- **Necrotizing Fasciitis:** "**Flesh-Eating** Streptococcus Disease"
  - Rapidly spreading gangrene of skin and fascia.
  - Starts as trivial skin infection but is **rapidly fatal**.
- **Pharyngitis:**
  - **Exudate on tonsils**, mostly in **children** (5-15 yrs old),.
- **Scarlet Fever (Scarlatina):**
  - **Red** maculopapular **"sandpaper" rash** on trunk, intense at **skinfolds**.
  - White and red **"strawberry tongue."**
  - Follows pharyngeal or other infections by strains which elaborate **erythrogenic toxin**.
- **Post-Streptococcal Acute Glomerular Nephritis (AGN):**
  - Non-suppurative sequelae. No Group A Streptococcus present.
  - **Post-pharyngitis** or **post-skin infection** (after infection resolves).
  - Symptoms: facial edema, blood in urine ("smoky" urine).
- **Post-Streptococcal Acute Rheumatic Fever (ARF):**
  - Non-suppurative sequelae. No Group A Streptococcus present.
  - **Post-pharyngitis only** (after infection resolves).
  - Symptoms: migratory **arthritis**, subcutaneous **nodules**, **carditis**, and erythema marginatum.
  - May proceed to **Rheumatic Heart Disease (RHD)**.

SOURCE & TRANSMISSION:
- **Normal flora** of **skin** and **oropharynx**.
- Causes infections upon penetration of tissues.

VIRULENCE FACTORS:
- **Exotoxins**
- **Protein M** (of cell wall): provides antigenic variation.
  - Blocks opsonization by complement alternate pathway, thus Group A Streptococcus evades phagocytosis.
- **Capsule:** resists phagocytosis
- **Hyaluronidase:** degrades hyaluronic acid in connective tissue.
- **Peptidase:** destroys C5a complement as a chemotactic signal to PMNs.
- **Streptokinase:** catalyzes activation of plasmin to lyse blood clots.
- Streptodornase (DNase): degrades DNA, provides antigenic variation.
- Pili, Lipoteichoic acid, and F-Protein: mediate attachment to epithelium.

TREATMENT:
- **Penicillin G**
- **Erythromycin** in Penicillin allergy
- Benzathine **Penicillin** prophylaxis to prevent recurrence of ARF.
- **Sulfonamides** prophylaxis for ARF in Penicillin allergy.
- Topical **Bacitracin**.

VACCINE & TOXOID:
None

HOST DEFENSE & IMMUNITY:
- IgA, IgM, IgG **antibodies** to M Protein offer resistance and **type specific immunity**, PMNs.
- **Autoimmunity** develops via cross reaction in **ARF**.
- **Immune complexes** involving C3 from complement alternate pathway deposited at glomerular BM in **AGN**
- **Serum C3** levels will be low in **AGN**
- Elevated **ASO titers** in **AGN** and **ARF**.

LAB TESTS:
- Catalase: Neg
- Hemolysis: **Beta**
- 6.5%NaCl: No growth
- CAMP Test   Neg
- Bile Esculin   Neg
- Lancefield: **Group A** (type of Carbohydrate C)
- **Bacitracin**   **Susceptible**

Streptococcus Group B (agalactiae)

GRAM STAIN:
POS

AEROBIC

EXTRACELLULAR

FEATURES:
- Cocci : Pairs, short chains.
- Colonies: gray-white
  on Blood-Agar.

MOTILITY:

None

CAPSULE & GLYCOCALYX:
- **Capsule:**
  Polysaccharide

EXOTOXINS:

None

CLINICAL:
- **Neonate Meningitis:**
  - Symptoms: **fever**, lethargy, poor feeding. Seizures = poor prognosis.
  - Invades via mucus membranes, respiratory tract, and sepsis; often **fatal**.
  - Meningitis must be diagnosed via **lumbar puncture**:
    CSF: ↑PMNs, ↓Glucose, Cloudy, Culture = GBS
  - **Early onset** (age 0-5 days):
  Vertical transmission in utero; ascending, due to ruptured amnionic sac.
  - **Late onset** (age 5-90 days):
  Vertical transmission at time of delivery; or can be nosocomial.
- **Neonate Pneumonia:**
  - Symptoms: cyanosis, tachypnea and respiratory distress, can be **fatal**.
  - **Early onset** only; via ascending vertical transmission.
- **Post-Partum Endometritis:**
  - Especially following C-Section.

SOURCE & TRANSMISSION:
- **Normal flora** of **vagina**.
- **Vertical transmission** either at birth or via ascension in utero.

VIRULENCE FACTORS:
- **Capsule**: type-specific polysaccharide, resists phagocytosis.
- **Sialic acid**: capsular component, inhibits alternate pathway of
  complement, especially type III strain.

TREATMENT:
- **Ampicillin plus aminoglycoside**
  for neonates.
- **Penicillin G** for adult.
- **Vancomycin** in Penicillin allergy.

VACCINE & TOXOID:

None

HOST DEFENSE & IMMUNITY:
- IgG Antibodies to capsule, PMNs.
- **Classic** path complement C1 activated by capsule, antibody-independent opsonization.
- **Alternate** path complement is involved in antibody-dependent opsonization.
- Note that neonate host defense is quickly defeated.

LAB TESTS:
- Catalase: Neg
- Hemolysis: **Beta**
- 6.5%NaCl: No growth
- **CAMP Test**   **Pos**
- Bile Esculin   Neg
- Lancefield: **Group B**
  (type of Carbohydrate C)

Streptococcus pneumoniae

GRAM STAIN:
POS

AEROBIC

EXTRACELLULAR

FEATURES:
- **Cocci** : Pairs.
- Colonies: gray-white, variable on Blood-Agar.

MOTILITY:
None

CAPSULE & GLYCOCALYX:
- **Capsule:**
  Polysaccharide
  80+ Types

EXOTOXINS:
None

CLINICAL:
- **Lobar Pneumonia:**
  (*S. pneumoniae* is #1 causative organism in **adults** and in sickle cell disease)
  - Symptoms: fever, cough with **sputum**, dull chest percussion, X-ray shows segmental consolidation. Can be **fatal**. Abscess is rare.
  - Diagnosis: based on presence of *S. pneumoniae* and PMNs in sputum.
  - Often predisposed by viral infection, alcoholism, smoking, or any condition which suppresses cough reflex or disrupts cilia.
- **Meningitis:**
  (*S. pneumoniae* is #1 causative organism in **adults** and **elderly**)
  - Symptoms: fever, neck pain, headache, POS **Brudzinski sign** and POS **Kernig sign**. Can be **fatal**.
  - Diagnosis: Lumbar puncture prior to antibiotic treatment: CSF: ↑PMNs, ↓Glucose, Cloudy, Culture.
  - Often follows sinusitis, otitis media, or bacteremia (via choroid plexus)
- **Sinusitis:** (*S. pneumoniae* is #1 causative organism).
  Often follows allergy or viral induced edema which prevents sinus drainage.
- **Otitis Media:** (*S. pneumoniae* is #1 causative organism).
  Often follows allergy or viral induced edema which prevents eustachian drainage.

SOURCE & TRANSMISSION:
- **Normal flora** of **upper respiratory tract**.
- **Pulmonary** infections occur when muccocilliary action fails. Alveoli get filled with bacteria which extend to entire lobe via pores of Kohn.
- **Meningitis** occurs from extension of sinusitis or otitis media, or from choroid seeding due to bacteremia.

VIRULENCE FACTORS:
- **Capsule:** enables *S. pneumoniae* to resist phagocytosis.
- **IgA protease:** prevents opsonization by IgA at mucus membranes.
- **Adhesins:** mediates attachment of *S. pneumoniae* to epithelial cells.

TREATMENT:
- **Penicillin G**
- **Vancomycin** in Penicillin allergy, but may be ineffective in meningitis.

VACCINE & TOXOID:
Vaccine made up of 23 capsular antigens.

HOST DEFENSE & IMMUNITY:
- **IgG Antibody** to capsule offers resistance and type specific immunity.
- **Classic** path complement C1 activated by capsule, antibody-independent opsonization.
- **Alternate** path complement is involved in antibody-dependent opsonization.
- **C5a** complement attracts **PMNs**.
- **Vaccine** confers immunity for a few years.

LAB TESTS:
- Catalase: Neg
- Hemolysis: **Alpha (green)**
- 6.5%NaCl: No growth
- CAMP Test   Neg
- Bile Esculin   Neg
- Lancefield: None
  (No Carbohydrate C)
- **Optochin   +/-Sensitive**
- **Bile Solubility Pos**

Streptococcus Group D

Streptococcus bovis and others

GRAM STAIN:
POS

AEROBIC

EXTRACELLULAR

FEATURES:
- **Cocci**: Pairs, chains
- Colonies: gray-white, variable on Blood-Agar.

MOTILITY:
None

CAPSULE & GLYCOCALYX:
Unknown

EXOTOXINS:
None

CLINICAL:
- **Bacteremia:**
  - *S. bovis* enters the blood via gastrointestinal route.
- **Sub-Acute Endocarditis:**
  - Arises from bacteremia. Can be **fatal** if untreated.
- **Colon Cancer:**
  - Strong association between *S. bovis* bacteremia and **colon cancer**. It is unknown which is cause or effect.

SOURCE & TRANSMISSION:
- **Normal flora** of **GI tract**.
- Causes infection upon entry into blood stream via GI tract.

VIRULENCE FACTORS:
None

TREATMENT:
- **Penicillin G**
- **Vancomycin** in Penicillin allergy

VACCINE & TOXOID:
None

HOST DEFENSE & IMMUNITY:
- IgA and IgG antibodies, PMNs.

LAB TESTS:
- Catalase: Neg
- **Hemolysis:** α or β or γ
- 6.5%NaCl: No growth
- CAMP Test: Neg
- **Bile Esculin** **Pos**
- Lancefield: **Group D** (type of Carbohydrate C)

Streptococcus Viridans Group

GRAM STAIN:
POS

Streptococcus mutans and others

AEROBIC

EXTRACELLULAR

FEATURES:
- Cocci : Pairs, chains
- Colonies: gray-white, variable on Blood-Agar.

MOTILITY:
None

CAPSULE & GLYCOCALYX:
- **Glycocalyx** only:
  Dextran

EXOTOXINS:
None

CLINICAL:
- **Sub-Acute Endocarditis**: (Number 1 causative organism).
  - Results from bacteremia, which follows recent dental work.
  - Infects only abnormal valves or prosthetic valves.
  - Can be **fatal** if untreated.
- **Dental Caries**.

SOURCE & TRANSMISSION:
- **Normal flora** of **oropharynx**.
- Causes infections when enters blood stream after dental work or due to poor oral hygiene.

VIRULENCE FACTORS:
- **Dextran** exopolysaccharide glycocalyx
  - Provides means of adherence to defective heart valves.
  - May block the action of antibiotics.
- **Lipoteichoic Acid** (LTA): mediates adhesion to fibronectin in clots on defective heart valves.
- **Glucans** are polysaccharides made by *S. mutans* from sucrose in mouth, they provide a means of attachment to tooth enamel
- **Acids**: are made by *S. mutans* from fermentation of sugars in mouth.

TREATMENT:
- **Penicillin G** plus **Aminoglycoside** must be given prophylactically before dental work or oral surgery to people with defective heart valves.
- **Vancomycin** in Penicillin allergy.

VACCINE & TOXOID:
None

HOST DEFENSE & IMMUNITY:
- Lysis of bacteria by serum enzymes and lysosomal enzymes.

LAB TESTS:
- Catalase: Neg
- Hemolysis: **Alpha (green)**
- 6.5%NaCl: No growth
- CAMP Test   Neg
- Bile Esculin   Neg
- Lancefield: **None**
  (No Carbohydrate C)
- **Optochin**   **Resistant**
- Bile Solubility Neg

Enterococcus spp formerly included in **Streptococcus** Group D

Enterococcus faecalis and others

GRAM STAIN:
POS

AEROBIC

EXTRACELLULAR

FEATURES:
- **Cocci** : Singly, pairs, chains
- Colonies: gray-white, variable on Blood-Agar.

MOTILITY:
None

CAPSULE & GLYCOCALYX:
Unknown

EXOTOXINS:
None

CLINICAL:
- **UTI:**
  - Upper (**pyelonephritis**) and lower (**cystitis**) urinary tract infections.
  - Most often **nosocomial**.
- **Bacteremia:**
  Via urinary tract infection, intra-abdominal infection, or nosocomial from various in-dwelling lines such as IV lines or during hemodialysis. Bacteremia may be predisposed by chronic illness or diabetes. Often **fatal.**
- **Sub-Acute Endocarditis**:
  - Results from bacteremia,
  - *Enterococcus* infects only **abnormal valves** or prosthetic valves.
  - **Fatal** if untreated.

SOURCE & TRANSMISSION:
- **Normal flora** of **GI tract**.
- Causes infection upon entry into blood stream.
- **Nosocomial:** exogenous acquisition of *Enterococcus* occurs often in hospitals.

VIRULENCE FACTORS:
- *Enterococcus* has a great ability to **resist antibiotics**.
- *Enterococcus* has the ability to **adhere to defective heart valves** and **urinary tract epithelial cells**.
- The mechanisms of virulence are **unknown**.

TREATMENT:
- **Vancomycin** plus **Aminoglycoside**
- **NOTE:** some Vancomycin-resistant strains of *Enterococcus* exist. In such cases there is no effective treatment.

VACCINE & TOXOID:
None

HOST DEFENSE & IMMUNITY:
Unknown.

LAB TESTS:
- Catalase: Neg
- **Hemolysis:**   α or β or γ
- **6.5%NaCl:**   **Growth**
- CAMP Test   Neg
- **Bile Esculin**   **Pos** (hydrolyzed)
- Lancefield: Group D (type of Carbohydrate C)

Chapter 3

GRAM POSITIVE RODS and Non-Commensal Anaerobes.

Bacillus cereus
  Food poisoning
  Eye infections

Corynebacterium diphtheriae
  Diphtheria
  Wound infections

ZOONOTIC GRAM POSITIVE RODS:

Listeria monocytogenes (Zoonotic)
  Abortion
  Meningitis
  Neonatal Granulomas

Bacillus anthracis (Zoonotic)
(see Zoonotic chapter)

NON-COMMENSAL ANAEROBES:

Clostridium botulinum (Anaerobic)
  Botulism food poisoning
    (flaccid paralysis)
  Infant botulism
  Wound botulism

Clostridium difficile (Anaerobic)
  Pseudomembranous colitis
    (post-antibiotic colitis)

Clostridium perfringens (Anaerobic)
  Gas gangrene
  Food poisoning
  GI necrosis

Clostridium tetani (Anaerobic)
  Tetanus wound infection
    (spastic paralysis)

OTHER GRAM POSITIVE RODS:

Actinomyces israelii (Anaerobic)
(see Commensal Anaerobe chapter)

Propionibacterium acnes (Anaerobic)
(see Commensal Anaerobe chapter)

Mycobacterium spp (Obligate Aerobic)
(see Gram Positive Acid Fast chapter)

Nocardia asteroides
(see Gram Positive Acid Fast chapter)

Bacillus cereus

GRAM STAIN:
POS

AEROBIC

EXTRACELLULAR

FEATURES:
- **Rods**: singly, pairs, chains.
- Colonies: granular appearance on nutrient agar, with the addition of certain amino acids.

MOTILITY:
Flagella

CAPSULE & GLYCOCALYX:
- **SPORES:**
Require oxygen.

EXOTOXINS:
- **Enterotoxins:**
  - Necrotic toxin: vascular permeability action.
  - Cereolysin: a hemolysin which disrupts cholesterol of cell membranes.

CLINICAL:
- **Emetic Food Poisoning:**
  - Symptoms: upper GI disturbance with **vomiting.**
  - *B. cereus* **spores** cool and germinate in **reheated rice**, especially in Chinese restaurant fried rice then grow rapidly before being ingested by host to cause symptoms.
  - Symptoms arise within **6 hours**.
  - Infection is self-limiting and lasts for a few hours.
- **Diarrheal Food Poisoning:**
  - Symptoms: lower GI disturbance with watery **diarrhea.**
  - *B. cereus* spores cool and germinate in **reheated meats or vegetables**, then grow rapidly before being ingested to cause symptoms.
  - Symptoms arise within **24 hours**.
  - Infection is self-limiting and lasts for one or two days.
- Eye infections: **post-traumatic endophthalmitis**, edema and ring abscesses. Occur especially among drug abusers. May cause blindness.

SOURCE & TRANSMISSION:
- **Spores** and *B. cereus* bacteria are found in **soil**, dust, decaying organic matter, and contaminated food.
- Non-invasive GI infection arises when bacteria are ingested.

VIRULENCE FACTORS:
- **Exotoxins**
- **Spore Formation:** enables survival in extreme and harsh conditions.
- Enzymes: lecithinase (phospholipase C) and others.

TREATMENT:
- Fluid and electrolyte replacement if necessary, but medication is not needed for food poisoning.
- **Vancomycin** for other infections.

VACCINE & TOXOID:
None

HOST DEFENSE & IMMUNITY:
Unknown.

LAB TESTS:
Not usually done.

Corynebacterium diphtheriae

GRAM STAIN:
POS

AEROBIC

EXTRACELLULAR

FEATURES:
●Rods: **Club**-shaped, has **granules**.
"V","L" or "**Chinese letter**" clumps
●Colonies: Dark gray or **black** on
potassium **Tellurite** medium.

MOTILITY:
None

CAPSULE & GLYCOCALYX:
None

EXOTOXINS:
●Diphtheria Toxin:
  ▪An **ADP-Ribosyltransferase**.
    Peptide B: binds to host cells to transport peptide A inside.
    Peptide A: has enzymatic activity.
  ▪Attaches ADP Ribose and prevents ribosome movement along mRNA.
  ▪Blocks host **EF2** (a protein synthesis elongation factor tRNA translocase).
  ▪**Blocks protein synthesis.**
  ▪Can kill host's NK cells (natural killer cells).
  ▪Coded on viral DNA which gets integrated into the bacteria by **lysogeny**
  (the process whereby a temperate Bacteriophage infects a bacterium).

CLINICAL:
●**Diphtheria:** (Rare in USA)
  ▪Symptoms: **Pseudomembrane** formation in throat: exudate forms a
    tough gray membrane which can lead to **stridor**, respiratory
    distress, cyanosis, lymphadenopathy. Can be **fatal**.
  ▪**Intoxication** consequences of diphtheria toxin:
    Cardiac Toxicity: occurs weeks after initial infection:
    Myocarditis, arrhythmias, A-V block. Can be **fatal**.
    Neurologic Toxicity: occurs only following severe infection:
    Early (first few days): **paralysis** of soft palate and pharynx.
    Late (months later): peripheral motor neuropathy.
  ▪Diagnosis must be made fast, and is based solely on symptoms.
●**Skin infections:** (Rare.)
  Infects open wound, mostly in persons with poor hygiene, in the tropics.
  Presents with gray membrane on non-healing wound.
●**Schick skin test:** (rarely performed): POS sign: red-brown spot appears at site
  of intradermal toxin injection after 36 hrs (therefore, patient is immune).

SOURCE & TRANSMISSION:
●**Humans** are the only reservoir for *C. diphtheria* upper
respiratory tract infections and skin lesions.
●Horizontal transmission occurs via **respiratory** droplets.

VIRULENCE FACTORS:
●Diphtheria exotoxin.
●Storage granules:
  ▪Contain phosphate polymers for high-energy reserve.
  ▪Stain with metachromatic dye (cell=blue, granules=red).

TREATMENT:
●**Penicillin G** to kill the organism.
●**Erythromycin** in Penicillin allergy
    to kill the organism.
●**Diphtheria Antitoxin**
(horse-derived **antibodies** to the toxin)
must be administered immediately.

VACCINE & TOXOID:
Toxoid: inactive toxin is
given as part of **DPT**

HOST DEFENSE & IMMUNITY:
●Antibodies develop to the toxin, but it is
usually too late to stop the toxic effects and
death
●Toxoid with boosters gives long-standing
immunity.
●The *C. diphtheria* is non-invasive so there
is no systemic infection.

LAB TESTS:
●Growth on **Loeffler** medium.
●**Metachromatic** staining of
    storage granules.
●Growth on **Tellurite** medium
yields **gray-black** colonies..

Listeria monocytogenes

GRAM STAIN:
POS

ZOONOTIC

AEROBIC

INTRACELLULAR

FEATURES:
- **Rods** : small, almost like cocci.
"**Chinese character**" clumps
- **Colonies:** translucent on
     Blood-Agar.

MOTILITY:
Tumble

CAPSULE & GLYCOCALYX:
None

EXOTOXINS:
- **Hemolysins:** (disrupt blood cells)
     - **Listeriolysin O:** mediates escape from phagolysosome.
          Enhanced by low pH and low iron (as found in lysosome).
          Acts by disrupting membranes (especially of the lysosome).

CLINICAL:
- **Abortion:**
     - Bacteremia can occur during pregnancy.
     - Mild fever for the mother.
     - Prematurely induces labor which may be **fatal** for the **fetus**.
- **Meningitis:**
     - **Neonatal Meningitis - Late onset** (age 5-90 days):
          Vertical transmission at time of delivery.
     - **Immunocompromised Meningitis:** elderly, cancer patients, and
          renal transplant patients.
     - Diagnosis: **Lumbar puncture** prior to antibiotic treatment:
          CSF: ↑PMNs, ↓Glucose, Cloudy, Culture.
- **Granulomatosis Infantiseptica:**
     - Neonatal **granulomas** and abscesses: skin, conjunctiva, organs, brain.
     - Results from **vertical transmission** either transplacental in utero or
          during birth.
     - Can be **fatal**.

SOURCE & TRANSMISSION:
- Animals are **zoonotic** reservoirs for *L. monocytogenes*, some
food products, especially **unpasteurized milk**, are sources.
- **Vertical transmission** occurs in utero via **transplacental**
infection or **during birth** due to passage through vagina.
- **Zoonotic** transmission occurs via contact with farm animals.

VIRULENCE FACTORS:
- **Hemolysin Listeriolysin O**
     - Enables *L. monocytogenes* to survive inside macrophages.

TREATMENT:
- **Penicillin G** or **Ampicillin**
- **TMP-SMZ** in Penicillin allergy.
- **Ampicillin plus Gentamicin** for
neonatal meningitis.
- **3rd Generation Cephalosporin.** in
penicillin and sulfa double allergy.

VACCINE & TOXOID:

None

HOST DEFENSE & IMMUNITY:
- T-cell mediated response plus Macros.

LAB TESTS:
- **Catalase:**   Pos
- **Hemolysis:**   Beta
- **Methyl Red**   Pos
- **Voges-Proskauer**   Pos
- **Bile Esculin**   Pos (hydrolyzed)

Clostridium botulinum

GRAM STAIN:
POS

OBLIGATE ANAEROBE

EXTRACELLULAR

FEATURES:
- Rods :
- Colonies: not usually cultured.

MOTILITY:
None

CAPSULE & GLYCOCALYX:
- **SPORES:**
killed at 80°C for 10 min.

EXOTOXINS:
- **Botulinum Toxin:**
  - **Preformed in food**.
  - 8 different types but types A, B, E cause human illness.
  - Heat labile at 121°C for 15 min.
  - **Neurotoxin**: one of the most potent toxins known.
    Blocks release of ACh (acetylcholine) from neurons.
    Causes **flaccid paralysis**.
  - Coded on viral DNA which gets integrated into the bacteria by **lysogeny** (the process whereby a temperate Bacteriophage infects a bacterium).

CLINICAL:
- **Botulism Food Poisoning:** (intoxication)
  - Caused by ingestion of **preformed toxin** in contaminated food.
    Note: no *C. botulinum* bacteria need to be ingested.
  - Symptoms: Early: nausea, vomit, diarrhea, with NO fever.
    Late: **Flaccid paralysis**, respiratory distress from diaphragm paralysis, can be **fatal** or take months-years to heal.
  - Diagnosis is made on basis of symptoms and history.
- **Infant Botulism:**
  - *C. botulinum* colonizes neonate colon as "normal" flora. Toxin is then produced to cause symptoms.
  - The source of *C. botulinum* in infant botulism is **honey**.
  - Symptoms: **feeble cry**, weakness, paralysis, respiratory distress.
    May account for **SIDS** (Sudden Infant Death Syndrome).
    Infant may spontaneously recover.
- **Wound Botulism:**
  - Spores enter wound, organisms grow and produce toxin.

SOURCE & TRANSMISSION:
- **Spores** occur in soil and in contaminated foods.
- Vacuum-packed canning enables the organism to grow from spores, and to produce toxin.
- Food poisoning occurs by ingesting **preformed toxin**.
- In infant botulism and wound botulism, the organism itself invades the host to cause colonization and infection.

VIRULENCE FACTORS:
- **Botulinum exotoxin**.
- **Spore Formation:** enables survival in extreme and harsh conditions.

TREATMENT:
- **Botulinum Antitoxin**
(horse-derived **antibodies** to the toxin)
- Respiratory support.
- **Prevention:** avoid bulging cans, boil or heat food well, avoid home-canning.
- Surgical wound debridement and **Metronidazole** for wound infection.

VACCINE & TOXOID:
None

HOST DEFENSE & IMMUNITY:
- Antibodies are ineffective.
- No immunity is gained by infection or intoxication.

LAB TESTS:
- Most labs can not detect toxin, and no tests are performed.

Clostridium difficile

GRAM STAIN:
POS

OBLIGATE ANAEROBE

EXTRACELLULAR

FEATURES:
- Rods
- Colonies:
  culture not usually done.

MOTILITY:
Peritrichous flagella

CAPSULE & GLYCOCALYX:
- SPORES:

EXOTOXINS:
- **Enterotoxin:**
  - **Toxin A:** agent of diarrhea and colitis
- **Cytotoxin:**
  - **Toxin B:** causes lysis of host cells, requires presence of Toxin A.

CLINICAL:
- **Antibiotic-Associate Colitis (AAC):** (*C. Difficile* is #1 causative organism)
  - Disease is also known as **"pseudomembranous colitis"**
  - **Nosocomial** and **iatrogenic:** most often arises within a few days of starting antibiotic therapy (especially **clindamycin**), especially in a newly hospitalized patient.
  - Symptoms: **explosive diarrhea** may be bloody and foul-smelling, fever, and yellow **pseudomembrane** formation in **colon**.
  - Antibiotics suppress commensal bacteria and enable the highly resistant *C. difficile* to flourish and produce toxins in abundance.
  - Diagnosis is made by stool sampling to detect concentration of **Toxins**. Colonoscopy is rarely done to see pseudomembrane.
  - Recurrence is possible.
  - Can be **fatal** in some cases if left untreated.

SOURCE & TRANSMISSION:
- The **spores** can survive on fomites and on surfaces in hospitals.
- *C. difficile* colonizes and outgrows commensal flora during the course of treatment with some antibiotics.

VIRULENCE FACTORS:
- **Exotoxins**
- *C. difficile* has a great ability to **resist many antibiotics**.
- **Spore Formation:** enables survival in extreme and harsh conditions.

TREATMENT:
- Continue current antibiotic treatment if possible.
- **IV Metronidazole**
- **oral Vancomycin** for serious infections.
- Electrolyte and fluid replacement may be necessary.

VACCINE & TOXOID:

None

HOST DEFENSE & IMMUNITY:
- Maintenance of normal colonic flora may prevent *C. difficile* colonization.

LAB TESTS:
- Tests are available to detect **toxin A or B** in **stool samples**.
- **CCFA media** (cycloserine, cefoxitin, and fructose agar) can be used to isolate the organism from stool samples.

Clostridium perfringens

GRAM STAIN:
POS

OBLIGATE ANAEROBE

EXTRACELLULAR

FEATURES:
- Rods: singly, pairs, chains
- Colonies: opaque, round: on blood agar, anaerobic conditions.

MOTILITY:

None

CAPSULE & GLYCOCALYX:
- SPORES:

EXOTOXINS:
- **Alpha Toxin:**
    - **Lecithinase:** hemolytic activity lyses membranes, including RBC and platelet membranes. **Necrotizing**.
- Beta Toxin, Epsilon toxin, Iota toxin: all are similar to Alpha toxin.
- Other minor toxins: many other toxins are expressed which have various enzymatic activities to promote necrosis of tissue.
- **Enterotoxin:** heat-labile agent of food poisoning.

CLINICAL:
- **Gas Gangrene:**
    - *C. perfringens* infection occurs mostly as a complication of surgery or trauma. **Spreads very rapidly** to cause local but spreading tissue necrosis and systemic intoxication. Can be rapidly **fatal**.
    - **Settings:** puncture wounds, GI tract surgery, burns or ischemic injury to skin or fascia, "back-alley" style abortions, war wounds, traffic accidents, and agricultural accidents.
    - **Alpha Toxin** causes **myonecrosis** (necrosis of skeletal muscle), gas is produced by *C. perfringens* fermentation of carbohydrates.
- **Food Poisoning:**
    - *C. perfringens* spores cool and germinate in previously heated food (mostly meats) then grow rapidly before being ingested by host to cause a very common but mild form of food poisoning and **diarrhea**.
    - **Enterotoxin** is released by *C. perfringens* in the small intestines to cause symptoms **within 7-15 hours**.
    - Infection is self-limited.
- **Enteritis Necroticans:**
    - Extremely rare Beta-Toxin induced GI-necrotizing infection.

SOURCE & TRANSMISSION:
- Spores occur in soil, dust, air.
- *C. perfringens* rarely, may be a part of normal intestinal flora.
- Disease occurs by entry of spores in wound site.

VIRULENCE FACTORS:
- **Exotoxins.**
- **Spore Formation:** enables survival in extreme and harsh conditions. Germination is enhanced by ischemic conditions.
- **Short generation time:** generation time of 10-12 minutes enables very rapid proliferation of *C. perfringens*

TREATMENT:
- Wound debridement or **amputation**, especially of muscle, on a daily basis until infection is under control.
- **Penicillin G** to kill the organism and for prophylaxis.
- **Metronidazole** in penicillin allergy, to kill the organism and for prophylaxis
- **Hyperbaric Oxygen**.

VACCINE & TOXOID:

None

HOST DEFENSE & IMMUNITY:
- Antibodies are most likely involved, but all host defenses seem to be ineffective against *C. perfringens* gas gangrene
- Antitoxin is no longer available because it was ineffective and caused allergic reactions.

So passive immunity is not available.

LAB TESTS:
- Blood agar colonies surrounded by **double zone beta hemolysis**.
- Milk media growth shows **stormy fermentation**.
- Egg yolk agar growth shows **lecithinase** production and ppt of insoluble diglycerides.

Clostridium tetani

GRAM STAIN:
POS

OBLIGATE ANAEROBE

EXTRACELLULAR

FEATURES:
- **Rods** :"**tennis racquet**" shaped; singly, pairs, chains
- Colonies: transparent, villous: on serum agar, anaerobic conditions.

MOTILITY:
Peritrichous flagella

CAPSULE & GLYCOCALYX:
- **SPORES:** killed at 121°C for 15 min. Carried along with the rod form.

EXOTOXINS:
- **Tetanus Toxin** (tetanospasmin):
  - Enters neuronal tissue by retrograde transport then **irreversibly** binds to block neurotransmitter release, **especially in GABA** and **GLY** pathways.
    B chain: binds to host cells to transport A chain inside.
    A chain: has enzymatic activity.
  - **Neurotoxin:**
    Blocks GABA and GLY inhibitory pathways, thus leaving the excitatory motor neurons un-opposed in a state of **tetany**
    This leads to **Spastic paralysis**.
  - Coded on a **Plasmid**.
- Hemolysin:
  Tetanolysin.

CLINICAL:
- **Wound infection: Tetanus** (lock-jaw):
  - *C. tetani* spores enter host via deep puncture wounds and dirty wounds, they germinate, grow and produce toxin.
  - **Tetanus toxin** blocks **GABA** and **GLY** inhibitory neural pathways, this leaves the excitatory motor neurons un-opposed in a state of tetany. This causes **Spastic paralysis** characterized by unremitting muscle contractions.
  - Symptoms:
  Note: Diagnosis must be made on basis of symptoms only.
    Trismus: lock-jaw
    Opisthotonos: whole body spasm with arched back and neck.
    Facial grimace.
    Respiratory distress occurs during spasms, can be **fatal**.
    Risus sardonicus: tetany of orbicularis oris.
  - **Transport of toxin** through neurons can take weeks, recovery may take months (if host survives), recurrence is possible.
  - Effects may remain localized to near the wound site.
- **Neonatal Tetanus:**
  - Due to infection of **umbilical stump**:
    (some cultures support using **mud** on stump).
  - Symptoms: baby will be weak, feverish, then rigid. **Mortality = 90%.**

SOURCE & TRANSMISSION:
- Spores occur in soil
- Disease occurs by entry of spores in wound site.

VIRULENCE FACTORS:
- **Tetanus exotoxin.**
- **Spore Formation:** enables survival in extreme and harsh conditions.

TREATMENT:
- **Tetanus Antitoxin:**
(human-derived **antibodies** to the toxin)
- **Diazepam** as a GABA-agonist.
- Respiratory support, and nutritional support.
- Surgical wound debridement.
- **Metronidazole** to kill the organism.

VACCINE & TOXOID:
Toxoid: inactive toxin is given as part of **DPT**

HOST DEFENSE & IMMUNITY:
- Antibodies develop to the toxin, but it is usually too late to stop the toxic effects and death
- Toxoid with boosters gives long-standing immunity.

LAB TESTS:
- No tests are usually performed.

Chapter 4

COMMENSAL ANAEROBIC BACTERIA

GRAM POSITIVE COCCI

Peptostreptococcus spp
> Soft-tissue abscess

GRAM POSITIVE RODS

Actinomyces israelii
> Oral Actinomycosis
> Lung Actinomycosis
> Pelvic Actinomycosis

Propionibacterium acnes
> Acne vulgaris

GRAM NEGATIVE RODS

Bacteroides fragilis
> Intra-abdominal abscess
> Peritonitis
> Bacteremia and Sepsis
> Female genital infections

Fusobacterium spp
> Odontogenic-Oral-Mandibular infections
> Chronic sinusitis
> Brain abscess
> Lung abscess
> Bacteremia and sepsis

Prevotella melaninogenica
> Periodontal disease
>> (gingivitis, trench mouth)
> Human bite wound infections
> Chronic sinusitis
> Brain abscess
> Lung abscess
> Bacteremia and sepsis
> Female genital infections

Peptostreptococcus spp

GRAM STAIN:
POS

OBLIGATE ANAEROBE

EXTRACELLULAR

FEATURES:
- Cocci
- Colonies: small white;
under **anaerobic** conditions,
on blood agar, or chocolate agar.

MOTILITY:

None

CAPSULE & GLYCOCALYX:
- **Capsule:**
Polysaccharide

EXOTOXINS:
None

CLINICAL:
- **Soft-Tissue Abscesses:**
  - Decubitus skin ulcers.
  - Diabetic foot ulcers.
  - Human bite wound infections.
  - Breast abscesses.
- May cause **bacteremia** and infect any organ of the body.

SOURCE & TRANSMISSION:
- *Peptostreptococcus* are very common commensal bacteria of
normal human **GI tract**, oral cavity, urogenital tract, and **skin**.
- Infection occurs via **endogenous spread** due to previous
surgery, immunocompromise, **diabetic** complications, etc.
- Infections with *Peptostreptococcus* are often **mixed** with other
anaerobes as well as aerobes in a powerful **synergy**.

VIRULENCE FACTORS:
- **Capsule:**
  - Enables *Peptostreptococcus* to resist phagocytosis.
  - Enhances abscess formation.
- *Peptostreptococcus* are low-virulent organisms that cause **opportunistic**
infections.

TREATMENT:
- **Penicillin G**
- **Vancomycin** in penicillin allergy.

VACCINE & TOXOID:

None

HOST DEFENSE & IMMUNITY:
- **IgM** and **IgG** antibodies to capsule are
important during sepsis.
- **Classic complement** pathway combined
with antibody, and **alternate** pathway, on its
own, are important for opsonization. **C5a** is
generated as a chemoattractant.
- **T-Cell** mediated immunity is important
during abscess.
- **PMN**'s are important during abscesses.

LAB TESTS:
- Culture.

Actinomyces israelii

GRAM STAIN:
POS

OBLIGATE ANAEROBE

EXTRACELLULAR

FEATURES:
- **Rods** : **Branching, filamentous.**
- Colonies: form **sulfur granules** in vivo. Grow slowly on many types of media (anaerobically).

MOTILITY:

None

CAPSULE & GLYCOCALYX:
- None.

EXOTOXINS:

None

CLINICAL:
- **Oral Actinomycosis** (cervical-facial):
  - Symptoms: **dental abscess** or painless soft tissue mass along jaw. Lesion arises from over growth of normal oral flora and may spread by direct extension to nearby structures. Lesion may open through skin to form a **sinus tract** which may contain purulent material mixed with yellow **sulfur granules.**
  - Presence of **sulfur granules** is pathopneumonic for *A. israelii* infection and of diagnostic value when combined with symptoms.
  - Do **not** confuse this disease with actinomycetoma which is caused by several aerobic bacteria (especially *Nocardia spp*) which are in the actinomycetes family. *A. israelii* does not cause mycetoma.
- **Lung Actinomycosis (Farmer's Lung):**
  - Symptoms: pneumonitis, chest pain, hemoptysis, empyema, fever.
  - X-ray may show mass lesion.
  - Infection was thought to arise from inhalation of spores present in grain but now is shown to arise from **aspiration** of the organism from the oral cavity. May extend to nearby structures.
- **Pelvic Actinomycosis:** rare, serious infection arising from long term IUD use.

SOURCE & TRANSMISSION:
- *A.israelii* is part of **normal dental flora**, and may be part of normal vaginal flora in some women.
- Infection arises during overgrowth of the organism due to poor hygiene, trauma, oral surgery, foreign body or due to aspiration.

VIRULENCE FACTORS:
- *A. israelii* is not very virulent and relies on groups of other bacteria to help get an infection started, therefore the actinomycosis infections are always **polymicrobial.**
- The "**sulfur granules**" are actually masses of the filamentous organism bound together with calcium phosphate.

TREATMENT:
- **Surgical debridement.**
- **Penicillin G** initially then **Amoxicillin** for one year to prevent recurrence.
- **Tetracycline** in penicillin allergy.
- **Erythromycin** in pregnancy and penicillin allergy.
- **Prevention:** good oral hygiene.

VACCINE & TOXOID:

None

HOST DEFENSE & IMMUNITY:
- Local, acute inflammation.

LAB TESTS:
- H&E stain of **sulfur granule** (which is a densely packed colony of *A. Israelii* found only in vivo) is eosinophilic.
- The branching chains of bacteria surround the granule, they can be visualized by using other stains or immunofluorescence.

Propionibacterium acnes

GRAM STAIN:
POS

OBLIGATE ANAEROBE

EXTRACELLULAR

FEATURES:
- **Rods** : sometimes **branching.**
- Colonies: grown anaerobically.

MOTILITY:
None

CAPSULE & GLYCOCALYX:
None

EXOTOXINS:

None

CLINICAL:
- **Acne Vulgaris (common acne):**
  - Chronic inflammatory infection of the pilosebaceous unit.
  - Infection occurs in papules, comedones (blackheads), pustules or cysts
  - Occurs mostly on the face, chest, shoulders, and back.
- **Bacteremia:** rarely associated with serious consequences.

SOURCE & TRANSMISSION:
- *P. acne* is part of **normal flora** of **skin**, mouth, eyes.
- Organism proliferates in acne lesions: it is not known if the infection is a cause of, or an effect of, the acne lesion.
- May enter blood via any puncture wound, needle stick, etc.

VIRULENCE FACTORS:
- *P. acne* has a great ability to stimulate the host's immune system to produce strong acute inflammation.

TREATMENT:
- **Benzoyl peroxide:** oxidizes the area for **topical** bacteriostatic effect.
- **Trimethoprim** for systemic treatment.
- **Retinoids** for cystic acne.

VACCINE & TOXOID:

None

HOST DEFENSE & IMMUNITY:
- *P. acne* releases substances which are chemotactic for **PMNs.**
- Activation of complement.

LAB TESTS:
- **Indole   Pos**
- Gas liquid chromatography reveals **propionic acid** as a metabolite of *P. acne*.
- *P. acne* frequently contaminates blood cultures due to its presence on skin.

Bacteroides fragilis

GRAM STAIN:
NEG

OBLIGATE ANAEROBE

EXTRACELLULAR

FEATURES:
- Rods : pale.
- Colonies: smooth, white-gray; under **anaerobic** conditions, on selective blood agar.

MOTILITY:
None

CAPSULE & GLYCOCALYX:
Capsule:
Polysaccharide.

EXOTOXINS:
None

ENDOTOXIN:

NOTE: Endotoxin of *B. fragilis* lacks lipid A, therefore it is **inactive**.

CLINICAL:
- **Intra-Abdominal Abscesses:** (#1 causative organism)
  - Occurs subsequent to **disruption of the colonic mucosa** due to any cause: trauma, **surgery**, ruptured appendix, or any **perforation**.
  - Most often found mixed with other anaerobes and aerobes; the aerobes initially consume local oxygen to enhance anaerobic growth.
- **Peritonitis:** (#1 causative organism)
  - Occurs subsequent to perforation of intestinal wall due to any cause.
- **Bacteremia and Sepsis:** (One of the most **common** causes of **bacteremia**)
  - *B. fragilis* most often spreads from an initial intra-abdominal infection.
  - Can lead to focal infections such as **endocarditis** and **brain abscesses.**
  - Symptoms: **fever** and prostration, but without septic shock (no lipid A). Very often **fatal**, especially if not treated effectively.
- **Genital Infections in Females:** occasional cause of pelvic abscesses and **PID**.

SOURCE & TRANSMISSION:
- *B. fragilis* is the **#1 commensal** bacteria of normal human **colon** (concentration 10^{11}/g feces), and sometimes **vagina**.
- Infection occurs via **endogenous spread** due to **perforation of bowel** or vagina due to any cause.
- Infections with *B. fragilis* are usually *mixed* with other anaerobes as well as aerobes in a powerful **synergy**.

VIRULENCE FACTORS:
- **Capsule:**
  - Enables *B. fragilis* to resist phagocytosis.
  - Enhances abscess formation.
- **Succinic Acid production:** enables *B. fragilis* to resist phagocytosis.
- **Enzymes:** promote tissue damage:
  - Collagenase, DNase, fibrinolysin, heparinase, hyaluronidase, and neuraminidase.
- **Catalase** and **Superoxide dismutase** enable *B. fragilis* to tolerate some oxygen and to escape phagocytic oxidative bursts.
- **β-Lactamase** coded on plasmid for β-lactam resistance.
- **Pili:** (Fimbria): mediates attachment to epithelial cells.
- Defective LPS is a poor chemoattractant.

TREATMENT:
- Surgical drainage of abscesses, along with debridement.
- **Metronidazole** for *B. fragilis* **plus 3rd Gen Cephalosporin** for mixed infections.
- **Hyperbaric Oxygen.**

VACCINE & TOXOID:

None

HOST DEFENSE & IMMUNITY:
- **IgM** and **IgG** antibodies to capsule are important during sepsis.
- **Classic complement** pathway combined with antibody, and **alternate** pathway on its own are important for opsonization. **C5a** is generated as a chemoattractant.
- **T-Cell** mediated immunity is important during abscess.
- **PMN**'s are important during abscesses.

LAB TESTS:
- Catalase   +/-
- Indole   +/-
- **20% Bile**   **Growth**
- **Colistin**   **Resistant**
- **Kanamycin**   **Resistant**
- **Vancomycin**   **Resistant**

Fusobacterium spp

GRAM STAIN:
NEG

OBLIGATE ANAEROBE

EXTRACELLULAR

FEATURES:
- **Rods** : long, thin, tapered ends.
- **Colonies:** irregular, "crumb-like;" under **anaerobic** conditions, on selective blood agar.

MOTILITY:
None

CAPSULE & GLYCOCALYX:
None

EXOTOXINS:
None

___

ENDOTOXIN:
- **Lipopolysaccharide** (LPS).

CLINICAL:
- **Odontogenic-Oral-Mandibular Infections:**
  - **Ludwigs Angina:** severe sub-maxillary and sub mandibular **cellulitis** spreading from **mandibular-molar** infection. Subsequent tongue elevation may lead to **strangulation.**
- **Chronic sinusitis** (more than three months): can directly extend to brain.
- **Brain Abscesses:** extension from sinusitis.
- **Lung Abscesses** and **Necrotizing Pneumonia:**
  - Infection follows aspiration of *Fusobacterium*
  - Infection sometimes arises from septic embolism from jugular vein.
  - <u>Symptoms</u>: **foul-smelling sputum,** cavitation, empyema.
- **Bacteremia and Sepsis:**
  - Most often spreads from an initial periodontal or lung infection.
  - Can lead to focal infections such as endocarditis and brain abscesses.
  - <u>Symptoms</u>: **fever** and prostration; can be **fatal** if not treated effectively.

SOURCE & TRANSMISSION:
- *Fusobacterium* are common **commensal** bacteria of normal human **gingiva.**
- Infection occurs via **endogenous overgrowth** within dental plaques due to **poor oral hygiene.** Aspiration occurs.
- Infections with *Fusobacterium* are usually *mixed* with other anaerobes as well as aerobes in a powerful **synergy.**

VIRULENCE FACTORS:
- **Endotoxin:** active.
- **Succinic Acid production:** enables resistance to phagocytosis.
- **Enzymes:** promote tissue damage:
  Collagenase, DNase, fibrinolysin, heparinase, hyaluronidase, neuraminidase, and phospholipase A.
- **Superoxide dismutase** enables *Fusobacterium* to escape phagocytic oxidative bursts.
- **β-Lactamase** coded on plasmid for β-lactam resistance.

TREATMENT:
- **Metronidazole** for *Fusobacterium* **plus 3rd Gen Cephalosporin** for mixed infections.
- **Good Oral Hygiene.**

VACCINE & TOXOID:
None

HOST DEFENSE & IMMUNITY:
- **IgM** and **IgG** antibodies to capsule are important during sepsis.
- **Classic complement** pathway combined with antibody, and **alternate** pathway on its own are important for opsonization. **C5a** is generated as a chemoattractant.
- **T-Cell** mediated immunity is important during abscess.
- **PMN's** are important during abscesses.

LAB TESTS:
- Catalase   Neg
- Indole   +/-
- 20% Bile   +/-
- Colistin   Sensitive
- Kanamycin   Sensitive
- **Vancomycin**   **Resistant**

Prevotella melaninogenica

GRAM STAIN:
NEG

OBLIGATE ANAEROBE

EXTRACELLULAR

FEATURES:
- **Rods** : pale.
- Colonies: **Brown**;
under **anaerobic** conditions,
on rabbit laked blood agar.

MOTILITY:
None

CAPSULE & GLYCOCALYX:
Capsule:
Polysaccharide.

EXOTOXINS:
None

ENDOTOXIN:
- **Lipopolysaccharide** (LPS).

CLINICAL:
- **Periodontal Disease:**
  - **Gingivitis:** bleeding **gums** and abscess formation, **halitosis**,
    loose teeth, and bone erosion.
  - **"Trench Mouth":** rare; acute necrotizing ulcerative gingivitis.
- **Human bite wound infection.**
- **Chronic sinusitis** (more than three months): can directly extend to brain.
- **Brain Abscesses:** extension from sinusitis.
- **Lung Abscesses and Necrotizing Pneumonia:**
  - Infection follows aspiration of *P. melaninogenica*
  - <u>Symptoms</u>: **foul-smelling sputum**, cavitation, empyema.
- **Bacteremia and Sepsis:**
  - Most often spreads from an initial periodontal or lung infection.
  - Can lead to focal infections such as endocarditis and brain abscesses.
  - <u>Symptoms</u>: **fever** and prostration; can be **fatal** if not treated effectively.
- **Genital Infections in Females:**
  - Common cause of **vaginosis** with foul-smelling vaginal discharge
  - Sometimes involved in **PID**.

SOURCE & TRANSMISSION:
- *P. melaninogenica* is the *#1 commensal* bacteria of normal human **gingiva** (concentration 10^{11}/ml); also common in **vagina**.
- Infection occurs via **endogenous overgrowth** within dental plaques and tonsils due to **poor oral hygiene**. Aspiration occurs.
- Infections with *P. melaninogenica* are usually *mixed* with other anaerobes as well as aerobes in a powerful **synergy**.

VIRULENCE FACTORS:
- **Endotoxin**
- **Capsule:**
  - Enables *P. melaninogenica* to resist phagocytosis.
  - Enhances abscess formation.
- **Succinic Acid production:** enables resistance to phagocytosis.
- **Enzymes:** promote tissue damage:
  Collagenase, DNase, fibrinolysin, heparinase, hyaluronidase, neuraminidase, and phospholipase A.
- **Superoxide dismutase** enables *P. melaninogenica* to escape phagocytic oxidative bursts.
- **β-Lactamase** coded on plasmid for β-lactam resistance.
- Growth is enhanced by **vitamin k** produced by concomitant bacteria.

TREATMENT:
- **Metronidazole** for *P. melaninogenica* plus **3rd Gen Cephalosporin** for mixed infections.
- **Good Oral Hygiene.**

VACCINE & TOXOID:
None

HOST DEFENSE & IMMUNITY:
- **IgM** and **IgG** antibodies to capsule are important during sepsis.
- **Classic complement** pathway combined with antibody, and **alternate** pathway on its own are important for opsonization. **C5a** is generated as a chemoattractant.
- **T-Cell** mediated immunity is important during abscess.
- **PMN**'s are important during abscesses.

LAB TESTS:
●Catalase	Neg
●Indole	+/-
●20% Bile	No Growth
●**Colistin**	**Resistant**
●Kanamycin	+/-
●Vancomycin	+/-
●**Pigmented:**	**Brown**
●**Red Fluorescence under UV**	

Chapter 5

GRAM NEGATIVE COCCI

Neisseria gonorrhoeae

       Sexually transmitted diseases
          Urethritis
          Endocervical infection
          PID
          Fitz-Hugh-Curtis Syndrome
       Neonatal purulent conjunctivitis
       Monarticular arthritis

Neisseria meningitidis

       Epidemic meningitis
       Meningococcemia
       Waterhouse-Friderichsen syndrome

Moraxella catarrhalis

       Otitis media

Neisseria gonorrhoeae

GRAM STAIN:
NEG

AEROBIC

INTRACELLULAR

FEATURES:
- Cocci Diplococci (pairs) with "**coffee bean**" appearance.
- Colonies: small, transparent or white on **chocolate agar**.

MOTILITY:
None

CAPSULE & GLYCOCALYX:
Capsule:
unknown material.

EXOTOXINS:
None.

ENDOTOXIN:
- **Lipooligosaccharide** (LOS):
  - May be released as membranes fragments into the extracellular space and may mediate joint problems in gonococcal arthritis.

CLINICAL:
- **Male STD:** site of infection may be urethral, anorectal, or pharyngeal depending on sexual practice, but urethral is most common.
  - **Urethritis:**
    - Symptoms: purulent discharge and dysuria begin within 7 days.
- **Female STD:** site of infection may be endocervical, anorectal, urethral, or vaginal, but endocervical is most common.
  - **Endocervical infection:**
    - Symptoms: purulent vaginal discharge, dysuria, pain, bleeding, but is often **asymptomatic** in women.
  - **Salpingitis**, **cervicitis**, **endometritis** and **PID**:
    - Result from an ascending infection and may cause **sterility** due to scarring of uterine tubes.
  - **Fitz-Hugh-Curtis Syndrome (Perihepatitis):**
    - Direct extension of infection from pelvis to **liver capsule**.
    - RUQ pain, laparoscopy will show "violin-string" adhesions.
- **Neonates:** Ophthalmia neonatorum: a purulent **conjunctivitis** which is acquired by the newborn at birth during passage through the birth canal.
- **Monoarticular Arthritis:**
  - *N. Gonorrhoeae* is #1 causative organism of teen/young adult arthritis.
  - Mostly of the knee, mostly in **females**.
  - Arises from *N. gonorrhoeae* **bacteremia**.
  - Associated with **HLA-B27** genotype.
- **Adult Conjunctivitis:** purulent, ulcerating, occurs due to autoinoculation.

SOURCE & TRANSMISSION:
- Humans are the only reservoir of *N. gonorrhoeae*.
- Horizontal transmission occurs via **sexual contact**.
- Autoinoculation brings infection to other parts of the body.
- **Vertical transmission** from mother to neonate **during birth**, occurs due to passage through infected vagina.
- **Deficiency of complement C5-C8** predisposes to bacteremia.

VIRULENCE FACTORS:
- **Endotoxin:** provides antigenic variation.
- **Capsule:** enables resistance to phagocytes, provides antigenic variation.
- **Pili:** mediates attachment to epithelial cells, provide antigenic variation.
- **IgA protease:** prevents opsonization by IgA on mucus membranes.
- **Surface Proteins** (provide serotype and antigenic variations):
  - Protein I (porin): forms hydrophilic pores in outer membrane.
  - Protein II (Opa): mediates adherence, found in opaque strains.
  - Protein III (Rmp): provides protection from antibodies.
- **β-Lactamase** coded on plasmid: for penicillin resistance.
- **Iron-binding protein:** binds iron needed by *N. gonorrhoeae* for its own metabolic processes.

TREATMENT:
- **Ceftriaxone**
- **Cefoxitin** plus **Doxycycline** during concurrent infection with *Chlamydia*
- **Spectinomycin**
for use in pregnancy with penicillin allergy; not for pharyngeal infection.
- **Condoms** and **sex education** for prevention.

VACCINE & TOXOID:

None

HOST DEFENSE & IMMUNITY:
- Once the columnar or cuboidal cells are penetrated by *N. gonorrhoeae*, there is a local acute inflammatory response with pus formation, activation of complement and many **PMNs**.

LAB TESTS:
- **Catalase**   Pos
- **Oxidase:**   Pos
- Sugar utilization reaction:
  - **Glucose** only.
- **PCR** or **LCR** tests may be used for identification in cases where culture is not possible.

Neisseria meningitidis

GRAM STAIN:
NEG

AEROBIC

INTRACELLULAR

FEATURES:
- **Cocci** Diplococci (pairs) with "**coffee bean**" appearance, tetrads.
- Colonies: small, transparent on **chocolate agar**.

MOTILITY:
None

CAPSULE & GLYCOCALYX:
Capsule:
Polysaccharide.

EXOTOXINS:
None.

ENDOTOXIN:
- **Lipooligosaccharide (LOS):**
  - *N. meningitidis* produces and sheds excessive amounts of **LOS** endotoxin as membrane fragments into the extracellular space.
  - **LOS** endotoxin stimulates the release of the cytokines TNFα and IL-1 this can then lead to hypotension and **septic shock**.

CLINICAL:
- **Epidemic Meningitis** (especially in **children**, **young adults**, and military):
  - Symptoms: fever, neck pain, headache, POS **Brudzinski sign** and POS **Kernig sign**. Can be **rapidly fatal**.
  - Diagnosis: Lumbar puncture prior to antibiotic treatment: CSF: ↑PMNs, ↓Glucose, Cloudy, Culture.
  - Follows **upper respiratory** infection or meningococcemia.
- **Meningococcemia** (Sepsis with *N. meningitidis*):
  - Symptoms: skin, mucus membranes and conjunctival rashes (blue/red petechia), weakness, hypotension, vascular collapse, shock.
  - **Rapidly fatal** in many cases.
  - Follows upper respiratory infection.
  - **Deficiency of complement C5-C8** predisposes to infection.
  - Petechia will worsen as infection progresses to **DIC**.
- **Waterhouse-Friderichsen Syndrome:**
  - Is a very fulminant form of *N. meningitidis* infection with rapid onset of **DIC**, bilateral **adrenal hemorrhage**, and coma. **Rapidly fatal**.

SOURCE & TRANSMISSION:
- Humans **carriers** are the only reservoir of *N. meningitidis*. The organism colonizes the **nasopharynx.**
- Horizontal transmission occurs via **respiratory droplets**.
- **Deficiency of complement C5-C8** predisposes to bacteremia.

VIRULENCE FACTORS:
- **Endotoxin:** provides antigenic variation and mediates **shock**.
- **Capsule:** enables resistance to phagocytes, provides antigenic variation.
- **Pili:** mediates attachment to **non-ciliated epithelial cells** of host.
- **IgA protease:** prevents opsonization by IgA on mucus membranes.
- **Surface Proteins:** provide antigenic variations.
- **Iron-scavenging protein:** scavenges iron from host stores (such as hemoglobin, transferrin, and lactoferrin of PMNs). Iron is needed by *N. meningitidis* for its own metabolic processes.

TREATMENT:
- **Penicillin G**
- **Chloramphenicol** in penicillin allergy. *x1 Cipro*
- **Rifampin prophylaxis** for contacts (household, schools, military, etc.), and for **carriers**.
- Hospitalization in **ICU isolation** is necessary for management of shock, DIC, and transmission of disease.

VACCINE & TOXOID:
Vaccine: polyvalent capsular antigens.

HOST DEFENSE & IMMUNITY:
- Circulating **antibodies** to capsule and activation of complement are important. PMNs abound in CSF.
- Antibodies can cross-react to other strains.
- Previous infection and vaccination confer long lasting immunity.
- Endotoxin stimulates **cytokines**: TNFα and IL-1 which may mediate **shock**.

LAB TESTS:
- **Catalase**   **Pos**
- **Oxidase:**   **Pos**
- Sugar utilization reaction: **Glucose** and **Maltose**.
- **Latex agglutination** of CSF for rapid diagnosis.
- **PCR** or **LCR** tests may be used for identification in cases where culture is not possible.

Moraxella catarrhalis

GRAM STAIN:
NEG

AEROBIC

EXTRACELLULAR

FEATURES:
- Cocci: **Diplococci** (pairs).
- Colonies: gray on **chocolate agar**.

MOTILITY:
None

CAPSULE & GLYCOCALYX:
Capsule:
Polysaccharide.

EXOTOXINS:
None

ENDOTOXIN:
- Lipopolysaccharide (LPS):

CLINICAL:
- **Otitis Media:**
  - *M. catarrhalis* commonly causes otitis media in **children**.
- Sinusitis
- Laryngitis
- Tracheitis
- Bacteremia in immunocompromised.

SOURCE & TRANSMISSION:
- Human **upper respiratory** tract and sometimes **vagina** are reservoirs for *M. catarrhalis*
- Causes infection upon penetration of tissues.
- Horizontal transmission occurs via **respiratory droplets**.
- Infects **children**, COPD patients, and immunocompromised.

VIRULENCE FACTORS:
- **Endotoxin:** provides antigenic variation and mediates **shock** .
- **Capsule:** enables resistance to phagocytes, provides antigenic variation.
- **Pili:** mediates attachment to **non-ciliated epithelial cells** of host.
- Enzymes.

TREATMENT:
- **Amoxicillin**
- **TMP-SMZ** in penicillin allergy.

VACCINE & TOXOID:

None

HOST DEFENSE & IMMUNITY:
- IgM, IgG, and IgA **antibodies** to capsule.

LAB TESTS:
- **Catalase**   Pos
- **Oxidase:**   Pos
- **DNase agar**   Pos
- Sugar utilization reaction :
        Sucrose only.

Chapter 6

GRAM NEGATIVE RODS Respiratory Related

Bordetella pertussis

Whooping cough

Haemophilus influenzae

Pneumonia
Meningitis
Epiglottitis
Sinusitis and otitis media
Purulent conjunctivitis

Klebsiella pneumoniae

Pneumonia
UTI
Bacteremia

Legionella pneumophila

Legionnaires' disease
(atypical pneumonia)
Pontiac fever

Pseudomonas aeruginosa

Pneumonia
Burn wound infections
Endocarditis in IV drug abusers
UTI
Bacteremia
Corneal Keratitis
External otitis ("swimmer's ears")

Bordetella pertussis

GRAM STAIN:
NEG

AEROBIC

EXTRACELLULAR

FEATURES:
- **Rods**: small, almost like cocci; singly, pairs, chains.
- **Colonies**: white, grow slow on Bordet-Gengou agar (4 days).

MOTILITY:
None

CAPSULE & GLYCOCALYX:
Capsule:
Polysaccharide.

EXOTOXINS:
- **Pertussis Toxin:**
  - **Deactivates inhibitory G-protein:** (turns **off** the **off signal**)
    5B-unit: binds to host cells to transport peptide A inside.
    A-unit: causes addition of ADP-Ribose to G_i-protein:
    ↑**adenylate cyclase**, causes ↑**cAMP**
  - Blocks PMN diapededis, binds fucosyl residue on PMNs to prevent binding to ELAM on endothelial cells.
  - Mediates binding to **ciliated epithelial cells**.
  - Activates pancreatic Islet cells.
- **Adenylate Cyclase Toxin:** adenylate cyclase activity, causes ↑**cAMP**:
  - Blocks chemotaxis and protects against phagocytosis, oxidative lysis
  - Stimulated by host's intracellular calmodulin, and causes local edema.
- Dermonecrotic Toxin: vascular smooth muscle contraction and ischemic necrosis
- Tracheal Toxin: Causes ciliastasis (blocks the protective movement of cilia).

ENDOTOXIN:
- **Lipopolysaccharide** (LPS):

CLINICAL:
- **Whooping cough:**
  - Symptoms: acute tracheobronchitis with **paroxysmal cough** characterized by bouts of repetitive coughing with occasional **inspiratory "whoop"** sound due to the **narrowed glottis**; cough produces copious **mucus** which contains dead epithelial cells.
  - Symptoms last 1 week to 1 month.
- **Complications of *B. pertussis* infection:**
  - Pneumonia from aspiration, can be **fatal**.
  - Physical injury from coughing.
  - CNS abnormalities and seizures due to venous congestion and pressure from coughing.
- **Complications from vaccination:**
  - Whole-dead-cell vaccine can cause encephalopathy on rare occasion.

SOURCE & TRANSMISSION:
- Humans are the only reservoir of *B. pertussis.*
- Horizontal transmission is via **respiratory droplets** mostly among **infants** and **children**.
- **Highly contagious**.

VIRULENCE FACTORS:
- **Exotoxins.**
- **Endotoxin.**
- **Capsule:** enables *B. pertussis* to withstand phagocytosis.
- **Filamentous hemagglutinin:** surface protein which mediates attachment to **ciliated epithelial cells**.

TREATMENT:
- **Erythromycin:** may prevent complications and reduce infectivity, but the disease will still run its course.
- Oxygen therapy or suction of mucus may be necessary in children.

VACCINE & TOXOID:
Vaccine: part of **DPT**: Killed bacteria.

HOST DEFENSE & IMMUNITY:
- IgA, IgM, IgG **antibodies** to the various cell surface components, capsule and toxins.
- Infection is **non-invasive**, it remains localized to the upper respiratory tract.
- Vaccine and previous infection confer long lasting **immunity** (boosters are not necessary because *B. pertussis* rarely infects adults).

LAB TESTS:
- **Oxidase:** Pos
- **DFA test:**
  (direct fluorescent antibody test) to identify *B. pertussis* in smear.
- **Agglutination reaction** with antiserum.

Haemophilus influenzae

GRAM STAIN:
NEG
BIPOLAR STAINING

"Type b *H. Influenzae*" (Hib)
"Non-Typeable *H. Influenzae*" (ntHi)

AEROBIC

EXTRACELLULAR

FEATURES:
- **Rods** : small, almost like cocci;
- **Colonies:** small, translucent and round. Growth requires presence of **Factors X (heme) and V (NAD)**.

MOTILITY:
None

CAPSULE & GLYCOCALYX:
Capsule:
Polysaccharide.

EXOTOXINS:
None.

ENDOTOXIN:
- **Lipopolysaccharide (LPS):**

CLINICAL:
- **Pneumonia** (especially in **young children** and **elderly**):
  - Symptoms: fever, cough with purulent sputum. Can be **fatal**.
  - Due to type b and ntHi strains.
  - Often predisposed by alcoholism, smoking, or COPD.
- **Meningitis:**
(*H. Influenzae* is #1 causative organism in **very young children**: 6 mos-6 yrs):
  - Symptoms: fever, neck pain, headache, weakness, **nuchal rigidity**. Can be **rapidly fatal**.
  - Diagnosis: Lumbar puncture prior to antibiotic treatment:
    CSF: ↑PMNs, ↓Glucose, Cloudy, Culture.
  - Follows **upper respiratory** infection by type b (rarely ntHi strain).
- **Epiglottitis:**
(*H. Influenzae* is #1 causative organism, especially in young children):
  - Symptoms: fever and sore throat rapidly progressing to dysphagia and drooling. **Rapidly fatal** (hrs) from airway obstruction. Due to type b
- **Sinusitis and Otitis Media:**
  - Mostly in children; due to ntHi strains .
- **Purulent Conjunctivitis:**
  - Can occur as an epidemic; due to ntHi strains; can be **fatal**.

SOURCE & TRANSMISSION:
- Humans are the only reservoir of *H. influenzae*
- Horizontal transmission of type b is via **respiratory droplets**.
- The non-encapsulated strain ntHi (nontypeable *H. influenzae*) is part of the normal flora of the pharynx and conjunctiva.

VIRULENCE FACTORS:
- Endotoxin.
- **Capsule:** enables *H. Influenzae* type b to withstand phagocytosis.
  - This polysaccharide capsule contains ribose, ribitol and phosphate; referred to as polyribitol phosphate (PRP).
  - Nontypeable *H. Influenzae* strain ntHi, has no capsule.
- **IgA protease:**
  - Prevents opsonization by IgA on mucus membranes.
- **β-Lactamase** coded on plasmid: for penicillin resistance.

TREATMENT:
- **Cefotaxime or ceftriaxone** for pneumonia or meningitis.
- **Intubation immediately** for epiglottitis.
- **Chloramphenicol** for all serious *H. influenzae* infections in penicillin allergy.
- **Rifampin** prophylaxis for contacts.

VACCINE & TOXOID:
Vaccine: polysaccharide conjugated to protien for type b

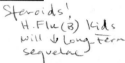
Steroids!
H. Flu (B) kids
will ↓ long term
sequelae

HOST DEFENSE & IMMUNITY:
- IgM, IgG **antibodies** to the PRP capsule.
- Infants lose maternal IgG within months.
- Activation of both classic and alternate paths of complement is important.
- PMNs and Macros respond, but Macros (especially in spleen) are most important.
- Vaccine confers immunity for a few years, boosters may be helpful.

LAB TESTS:
- May be grown on **blood agar** when *S. aureus* is present: *S. aureus* provides factor V, and blood agar provides factor X.
- **Catalase   Pos**
- Fermentation of **glucose** only.

Klebsiella pneumoniae

GRAM STAIN:
NEG

AEROBIC

EXTRACELLULAR

FEATURES:
- **Rods** : large and long.
- Colonies: large, **slimy**, mucoid, and white on blood agar.

MOTILITY:
None

CAPSULE & GLYCOCALYX:
Large Capsule:
Polysaccharide.

EXOTOXINS:
None.

___

ENDOTOXIN:
- **Lipopolysaccharide** (LPS):

CLINICAL:
- **Pneumonia:**
  - Bronchopneumonia and **Lobar pneumonia.**
  - Symptoms: fever, cough, empyema and hemoptysis with the formation of **thick "currant jelly' sputum.**
  - **Abscess formation** is common. **Can be fatal.**
  - X-ray shows "bowed fissure" infiltrated lower lobe.
  - Nosocomial acquired or community acquired in patients with alcoholism, diabetes mellitus or COPD.
- **UTI:**
  - *K. pneumoniae* is a very common cause of nosocomially acquired urinary tract infections.
- **Bacteremia:**
  - *K. pneumoniae* is second only to *E. coli* as a cause of nosocomially acquired bacteremia.

SOURCE & TRANSMISSION:
- *K. pneumoniae* can be part of the normal flora of the **colon.**
- **Nosocomial** transmission occurs via in-dwelling catheters and endotracheal tubes.

VIRULENCE FACTORS:
- Endotoxin.
- **Capsule:** enables *K. pneumoniae* to withstand phagocytosis.
- **β-Lactamase** coded on R-plasmid for β-lactam resistance and aminoglycoside resistance.
- **Urease** may help mediate the development of UTIs.

TREATMENT:
- Treatment requires the use of **multiple antibiotics:**
3rd generation cephalosporin plus aminoglycoside would be first choice, such as **cefotaxime plus gentamicin.**
- **TMP-SMZ** in penicillin allergy.

VACCINE & TOXOID:

None

HOST DEFENSE & IMMUNITY:
- Antibodies against capsule and LPS.

LAB TESTS:
- Oxidase   Neg
- **Lactose**   **Pos**
(Pink colonies on MacConkey)
- Indole   Neg
- Methyl red   Neg
- **Voges-Proskauer**   **Pos**
- **Simmon's citrate**   **Pos**
- TSI (H2S)   Neg
- **Urease**   **Pos**
- Fermentation of **glucose, sucrose** and **lactose.**

Legionella pneumophila

GRAM STAIN:
NEG

AEROBIC

INTRACELLULAR

FEATURES:
- **Rods**: thin
- **Colonies**: slow growth (5 days) on buffered charcoal yeast extract (BCYE) with cysteine and iron.

MOTILITY:
Mono-trichous flagella

CAPSULE & GLYCOCALYX:
None.

EXOTOXINS:
- *L. pneumophilia* releases some toxins which may mediate its ability to proliferate within alveolar macrophages.

ENDOTOXIN:
- **Lipopolysaccharide** (LPS):

CLINICAL:
- **Legionnaires' Disease:**
  - **Atypical pneumonia**.
  - <u>Symptoms</u>: **non-productive cough** and fever develops within 7 days.
  - X-ray usually shows unilateral, lower lobe involvement.
  - May be **fatal in the elderly and immunocompromised** patients, otherwise may resolve spontaneously.
  - Nosocomial or community acquired.
- **Pontiac fever:**
  - <u>Symptoms</u>: fever, chills, headache and sometimes nausea develop within 48 hours and spontaneously resolve within 1 week.

SOURCE & TRANSMISSION:
- **Air conditioners**, **whirlpool baths**, **humidifiers**, and **contaminated water** supply systems can be reservoirs for *L. pneumophilia* both in hospitals and in community settings.
- Transmission occurs by **inhalation of aerosols**, by **aspiration** of contaminated water, but **not** from person to person.

VIRULENCE FACTORS:
- Endotoxin.
- *L. pneumophilia* has a great ability to **prevent the fusion of the phagolysosome** when it is ingested by alveolar macrophages or blood monocytes. This enables the organism to proliferate within these cells.
- **Proteolytic enzymes** (proteases, esterases, phosphatases, endonucleases and peptidases) are produced to lyse the host macros and monos. This becomes a cycle of ingestion, proliferation, then escape by lysis.
- **β-Lactamase** coded on plasmid: for penicillin resistance.

TREATMENT:
- **Erythromycin** or other macrolide.
- **Prevention:**
super-hot water flushing of water supply and use of UV light is effective, but chlorination is not.

VACCINE & TOXOID:
None

HOST DEFENSE & IMMUNITY:
- Antibodies and complement are ineffective to opsonize the organism.
- **T-cell mediated** immunity is the best host defense against *L. pneumophilia*.

LAB TESTS:
- Produces **brown** pigment.
- **Catalase**　　**Pos**
- DFA test:
    Direct IFA stain of specimen
- Urinary Antigen test.

Pseudomonas aeruginosa

GRAM STAIN:
NEG

OBLIGATE AEROBE

EXTRACELLULAR

FEATURES:
- **Rods**: Long and thin; occur singly, pairs, chains.
- **Colonies**: large; on nutrient agar; **blue green color** and **fruity odor**.

MOTILITY:
Mono-trichous flagella

CAPSULE & GLYCOCALYX:
Glycocalyx:
Exopolysaccharide.

EXOTOXINS:
- **Exotoxin A** (diphtheria-like toxin):
  - An **ADP-Ribosyltransferase**.
    - **Peptide B**: binds to host cells to transport peptide A inside.
    - **Peptide A**: has enzymatic activity.
  - Attaches ADP Ribose and prevents ribosome movement along mRNA.
  - Blocks host **EF2** (a protein synthesis elongation factor tRNA translocase).
  - **Blocks protein synthesis.**
  - Mediates local necrosis and systemic spread of infection.
- **Exoenzyme S** (similar to exotoxin A):
  - May specifically mediate burn wound and lung infections.
  - Mediates attachment to host cells and suppression of immune response.
- **Hemolysins** (disrupt membrane lipids):
  - **Phospholipase C:**
    - Degrades phosphatidylcholine of surfactant to cause **atelectasis**.
  - **Rhamnolipid:** may inhibit mucociliary action in respiratory system.

ENDOTOXIN:
- **Lipopolysaccharide** (LPS): mediates **septic shock**.

CLINICAL:
- **Pneumonia** (necrotizing bronchopneumonia):
  - **Symptoms**: fever, cough, purulent sputum, cyanosis, lung abscesses.
  - **X-ray** may show bilateral nodularity and cavitation in lower lobes.
  - Infection arises either from aspiration after pharyngeal colonization, or secondarily from seeding of lung tissue during bacteremia.
  - Occurs in **immunocompromised**, COPD or **cystic fibrosis** patients.
  - Mostly **nosocomially acquired**. Mostly fulminant and **rapidly fatal**.
- **Burn Wound Infection:**
  - Black or **blue-green discoloration** of the wound; strong **fruity odor**.
  - May rapidly progress to cause necrosis of adjacent healthy tissue and to cause serious systemic infection. Can be **fatal**.
  - Mostly **nosocomially acquired**; especially in burn treatment units.
- **Endocarditis** (acute or subacute) in **IV drug users**:
  - Mostly effects the right heart, especially the tricuspid valve.
- **UTI**: nosocomially acquired; often iatrogenic, especially from catheterization.
- **Bacteremia**: in immunocompromised; can lead to septic shock; can be **fatal**. *P. aeruginosa* bacteremia can give rise to infection almost anywhere in the body.
- **Corneal Keratitis**: especially from **contact lens** use; can cause **blindness**.
- **Otitis Externa** ("Swimmer's ear"): may be benign or serious; often recurrent.

SOURCE & TRANSMISSION:
- *P. aeruginosa* is **everywhere**, especially in **moist areas** such as **hospital** sinks and respiratory equipment, swimming pools, whirlpool baths, raw vegetables, and human skin or mucosa.
- **Initial colonization** of **skin** or **mucosal surfaces** is required before the organism can spread to cause disease.

VIRULENCE FACTORS:
- **Endotoxin.**
- **Exotoxins.**
- **Glycocalyx:** enables *P. aeruginosa* to adhere to each other and to host epithelial cells. Also enables resistance to opsonization and phagocytosis.
- **Proteolytic enzymes** (elastase, protease, and others):
  - **Elastase:** cleaves IgA and IgG, cleaves complement, causes inactivation of TNFα and IFNγ, causes necrosis, disrupts the respiratory epithelium and inactivates the mucociliary action.
- **Pyocyanin:** a blue pigment which also mediates the formation of hydroxyl radicals and stimulates PMNs to damage host cells.
- **Multiple drug resistance:**
  - **β-Lactamase** coded on plasmid for β-lactam resistance.
  - **Acetylating enzymes** for aminoglycoside resistance.
  - **Mutant DNA gyrase** for fluoroquinolone resistance.
  - **Acetyltransferase** to break down chloramphenicol.

TREATMENT:
- Treatment requires the use of **multiple antibiotics:** first choice may be **gentamicin plus ticarcillin**
- **Aztreonam** in penicillin allergy.
- Treatment must be tailored to the specific strain of *P. aeruginosa*.
- Prevention of burn wound infection requires daily **wound debridement** and use of topical **silver sulfadiazine** (avoid hydrotherapy in bad burns).

VACCINE & TOXOID:

None

HOST DEFENSE & IMMUNITY:
- In general, immune-competent people have no trouble fighting *P. aeruginosa*.
- **Natural immunity**, such as intact skin and mucus membranes, is very important.
- Fully functioning IgM and IgG antibodies, classic and alternate complement, and PMNs are all necessary to fight and clear systemic infections of *P. aeruginosa*.

LAB TESTS:
- **Oxidase**   Pos
- **TSI** (H2S)   Neg
- **Simmon's citrate** Pos
- *P. aeruginosa* colonies produce **pigments** which blend into the culture medium:
  - **blue** (pyocyanin)
  - **green** (pyoverdin)
- *P. aeruginosa* colonies produce a **fruity odor**.

Chapter 7

GRAM NEGATIVE RODS Urinary Tract Related

Proteus mirabilis
>UTI
>Urolithiasis

Proteus vulgaris
Morganella morganii
Providencia rettgeri
>UTI
>Urolithiasis

Providencia stuartii
>UTI
>Bacteremia in nursing homes

Enterobacter cloacae
>UTI
>Bacteremia
>Opportunistic pneumonia

Serratia marcescens
>UTI
>Bacteremia
>Opportunistic Pneumonia
>Endocarditis in IV drug abusers
>Infective arthritis

Klebsiella pneumoniae
(see Gram Negative Rods Respiratory Related chapter)

Pseudomonas aeruginosa
(see Gram Negative Rods Respiratory Related chapter)

Uropathogenic Escherichia coli
>UTI
>Bacteremia
>Sepsis
>Opportunistic pneumonia
>Neonatal meningitis

Proteus mirabilis

GRAM STAIN:
NEG

AEROBIC

EXTRACELLULAR

FEATURES:
- **Rods** : singly, pairs, chains.
- Colonies: **swarm** on blood agar. May give off **putrid odor.**

MOTILITY:
Peritrichous flagella

CAPSULE & GLYCOCALYX:
None

EXOTOXINS:
None.

ENDOTOXIN:
- **Lipopolysaccharide** (LPS):

CLINICAL:
- **UTI** :
  - Upper (**pyelonephritis**) and lower (**cystitis**) urinary tract infections.
  - Symptoms:
    - **Pyelonephritis**: flank pain, **fever**, dysuria, ±cystitis symptoms.
    - **Cystitis**: dysuria, pyuria, ↑frequency, ↑urgency, ±hematuria.
  - Diagnosis: urine culture: >10^5 bacteria/ml.
  - *P. mirabilis* is a very common causative organism of UTI.
  - Mostly **community acquired**, but may be nosocomial.
  - Infections may be **acute** or **chronic**.
- **Nephrolithiasis** (aka Urolithiasis or Kidney stone formation):
  - **"Struvite stones"** aka **"Staghorn calculus"** are large stones formed in the renal pelvis due to the precipitation of magnesium-ammonium phosphate salts ("triple phosphate salts").
    - *Proteus* secretes **urease** which splits urea to generate **alkaline urine** which enables the precipitation of these salts.
  - The stones **obstruct urine flow** and promote persistence of UTI.
  - Urine sediment microscopy shows:
    characteristic "coffin lid" crystal:

SOURCE & TRANSMISSION:
- *Proteus* is often normal flora of the **colon**, but is also found in soil and water.
- Infection arises via **autoinoculation** (**fecal** contamination of the urethra), or **nosocomial** due to urinary catheterization.
- Horizontal transmission is common due to lack of hand washing.

VIRULENCE FACTORS:
- Endotoxin.
- **Urease:**
  - Splits urea to ammonium hydroxide; this creates alkaline urine.
  - **Alkaline urine** promotes precipitation of salts to form stones.
  - These **"struvite"** stones **obstruct urine flow** and promote epithelial cell destruction and persistent infection.
- **Strong motility.**

TREATMENT:
- **Ampicillin** for cystitis.
- **TMP-SMZ** for pyelonephritis, or for cystitis in penicillin allergy.

VACCINE & TOXOID:

None

HOST DEFENSE & IMMUNITY:
- IgA, IgM, IgG **antibodies** to various cell surface components.
- **PMNs** respond in **acute** infections.
- **Macros** and **lymphocytes** respond in **chronic** infections.

LAB TESTS:
Oxidase	Neg
Lactose	Neg
Indole	Neg
Methyl Red	**Pos**
Voges-Proskauer	Neg
Simmon's citrate	**Pos**
TSI (H$_2$S)	**Pos**
Urease	**Pos**

Proteus vulgaris
Morganella morganii
Providencia rettgeri

GRAM STAIN:
NEG

AEROBIC

EXTRACELLULAR

FEATURES:
- **Rods** : singly, pairs, chains.
- Colonies: **swarm** on blood agar. May give off **putrid odor**.

MOTILITY:
Peritrichous flagella

CAPSULE & GLYCOCALYX:
None

EXOTOXINS:
None.

ENDOTOXIN:
- **Lipopolysaccharide** (LPS):

CLINICAL:
- **UTI :**
  - ▪ Upper (**pyelonephritis**) and lower (**cystitis**) urinary tract infections.
  - ▪ Symptoms:
    - **Pyelonephritis**: flank pain, **fever**, dysuria, ±cystitis symptoms.
    - **Cystitis**: dysuria, pyuria, ↑frequency, ↑urgency, ±hematuria.
  - ▪ Diagnosis: urine culture: >10^5 bacteria/ml.
  - ▪ Mostly **nosocomially acquired**.
  - ▪ These are **opportunistic** infections in the **immunocompromised**.
  - ▪ Infections may be **acute** or **chronic**.
- **Nephrolithiasis** (aka Urolithiasis or Kidney stone formation):
  - ▪ "**Struvite stones**" aka "**Staghorn calculus**" are large stones formed in the renal pelvis due to the precipitation of magnesium-ammonium phosphate salts ("triple phosphate salts"). *Proteus* secretes **urease** which splits urea to generate **alkaline urine** which enables the precipitation of these salts.
  - ▪ The stones **obstruct urine flow** and promote persistence of UTI.
  - ▪ Urine sediment microscopy shows: characteristic "coffin lid" crystal:

SOURCE & TRANSMISSION:
- These bacteria are often normal flora of the **colon**, but are also found in soil and water.
- Transmission is mostly **nosocomial** via **urinary catheter**. This occurs as an **opportunistic** infection in immunocompromised or otherwise debilitated patients.
- Horizontal transmission is common due to lack of hand washing.

VIRULENCE FACTORS:
- Endotoxin.
- **Urease:**
  - ▪ Splits urea to ammonium hydroxide; this creates alkaline urine.
  - ▪ **Alkaline urine** promotes precipitation of salts to form stones.
  - ▪ These "**struvite**" stones **obstruct urine flow** and promote epithelial cell destruction and persistent infection.
- **Strong motility.**
- **Multiple antibiotic resistance.**

TREATMENT:
- **Ampicillin** for cystitis.
- **TMP-SMZ** for pyelonephritis, or for cystitis in penicillin allergy.
- **Amikacin** for resistant strains.

VACCINE & TOXOID:

None

HOST DEFENSE & IMMUNITY:
- In general, immune-competent people have no trouble fighting these bacteria.
- IgA, IgM, IgG **antibodies** to various cell surface components.
- **PMNs** respond in **acute** infections.
- **Macros** and **lymphocytes** respond in **chronic** infections.

LAB TESTS:
● Oxidase	Neg
● Lactose	Neg
● **Indole**	**Pos**
● **Methyl Red**	**Pos**
● Voges-Proskauer	Neg
● Simmon's citrate	+/-
● TSI (H_2S)	+/-
● **Urease**	**Pos**

Providencia stuartii

GRAM STAIN:
NEG

AEROBIC

EXTRACELLULAR

FEATURES:
● **Rods** : singly, pairs, chains.
● Colonies: on blood agar.

MOTILITY:
Peritrichous flagella

CAPSULE & GLYCOCALYX:
None

EXOTOXINS:
None.

ENDOTOXIN:
● **Lipopolysaccharide** (LPS): mediates septic shock.

CLINICAL:
● **UTI :**
 ▪ Upper (**pyelonephritis**) and lower (**cystitis**) urinary tract infections.
 ▪ Symptoms:
  Pyelonephritis: flank pain, **fever**, dysuria, ±cystitis symptoms.
  Cystitis: dysuria, pyuria, ↑frequency, ↑urgency, ±hematuria.
 ▪ Diagnosis: urine culture: >10^5 bacteria/ml.
 ▪ Mostly **nosocomially acquired**.
 ▪ These are **opportunistic** infections in the **immunocompromised**.
 ▪ Infections may be **acute** or **chronic**.
● **Bacteremia:**
 ▪ *P. stuartii* is a very common causative organism of **nosocomial** bacteremia in **nursing home** patients with **chronic catheterization**.

SOURCE & TRANSMISSION:
● These bacteria are often normal flora of the **colon**, but are also found in soil and water.
● Transmission is mostly **nosocomial** via **urinary catheter**. This occurs as an **opportunistic** infection in immunocompromised or otherwise debilitated patients.
● Horizontal transmission is common due to lack of hand washing.

VIRULENCE FACTORS:
● **Endotoxin**.
● **Strong motility**.
● **Multiple antibiotic resistance**.

TREATMENT:
● **Ampicillin** for cystitis.
● **TMP-SMZ** for pyelonephritis, or for cystitis in penicillin allergy.
● **Amikacin** for resistant strains.

VACCINE & TOXOID:
None

HOST DEFENSE & IMMUNITY:
● In general, immune-competent people have no trouble fighting *P. stuartii*.
● IgA, IgM, IgG **antibodies** to various cell surface components.
● **PMNs** respond in **acute** infections.
● **Macros** and **lymphocytes** respond in **chronic** infections.

LAB TESTS:
● Oxidase	Neg
● Lactose	Neg
● **Indole**	**Pos**
● **Methyl Red**	**Pos**
● Voges-Proskauer	Neg
● Simmon's citrate	+/-
● TSI (H_2S)	+/-
● Urease	Neg

Enterobacter cloacae

GRAM STAIN:
NEG

AEROBIC

EXTRACELLULAR

FEATURES:
- **Rods** : singly.
- **Colonies**: white, may be mucoid; on blood agar.

MOTILITY:
Flagella

CAPSULE & GLYCOCALYX:
Capsule: small or absent, Polysaccharide

EXOTOXINS:
None.

ENDOTOXIN:
- **Lipopolysaccharide** (LPS): mediates septic shock.

CLINICAL:
- **UTI** :
  - Upper (**pyelonephritis**) and lower (**cystitis**) urinary tract infections.
  - Symptoms:
    - **Pyelonephritis**: flank pain, **fever**, dysuria, ±cystitis symptoms.
    - **Cystitis**: dysuria, pyuria, ↑frequency, ↑urgency, ±hematuria.
  - Diagnosis: urine culture: $>10^5$ bacteria/ml.
  - Mostly **nosocomially acquired**.
  - These are **opportunistic** infections in the **immunocompromised**.
  - Infections may be **acute** or **chronic**.
- **Bacteremia:**
  - As a complication of UTI, pneumonia, IV lines or IV injections.
- **Pneumonia:**
  - Mostly **nosocomially acquired**.
  - These are **opportunistic** infections in the **immunocompromised**.

SOURCE & TRANSMISSION:
- These bacteria are often normal flora of the **colon**.
- Transmission is mostly **nosocomial** via **urinary catheter**, or via respiratory equipment. This occurs as an **opportunistic** infection in immunocompromised or otherwise debilitated patients.
- Horizontal transmission is common due to lack of hand washing.

VIRULENCE FACTORS:
- **Endotoxin**.
- **Multiple antibiotic resistance**.

TREATMENT:
- **Ampicillin** for cystitis.
- **TMP-SMZ** for pyelonephritis, or for cystitis in penicillin allergy.
- **Amikacin** for resistant strains.

VACCINE & TOXOID:

None

HOST DEFENSE & IMMUNITY:
- In general, immune-competent people have no trouble fighting *E. cloacae*
- IgA, IgM, IgG **antibodies** to various cell surface components.
- **PMNs** respond in **acute** infections.
- **Macros** and **lymphocytes** respond in **chronic** infections.

LAB TESTS:
Oxidase	Neg
Lactose	**Pos**
(Pink colonies on MacConkey)	
Indole	Neg
Methyl Red	Neg
Voges-Proskauer	**Pos**
Simmon's citrate	**Pos**
TSI (H$_2$S)	Neg
Urease	+/-

Serratia marcescens

GRAM STAIN:
NEG

AEROBIC

EXTRACELLULAR

FEATURES:
- **Rods** : singly.
- Colonies: large white or red; on DNA agar

MOTILITY:
Flagella

CAPSULE & GLYCOCALYX:
None

EXOTOXINS:
None.

ENDOTOXIN:
- **Lipopolysaccharide** (LPS): mediates septic shock.

CLINICAL:
- **UTI :**
  - Upper (**pyelonephritis**) and lower (**cystitis**) urinary tract infections.
  - Symptoms:
    Pyelonephritis: flank pain, **fever**, dysuria, ±cystitis symptoms.
    Cystitis: dysuria, pyuria, ↑frequency, ↑urgency, ±hematuria.
  - Diagnosis: urine culture: $>10^5$ bacteria/ml.
  - Mostly **nosocomially acquired**.
  - These are **opportunistic** infections in the **immunocompromised**.
  - Infections may be **acute** or **chronic**.
- **Bacteremia:**
  - As a complication of UTI, pneumonia, IV lines or IV injections.
- **Pneumonia:**
  - Mostly **nosocomially acquired**.
  - These are **opportunistic** infections in the **immunocompromised**.
- **Endocarditis** in **IV drug users** (heroin):
  - Mostly effects the **right heart**, especially the **tricuspid** valve.
- **Infective Arthritis:**
  - Iatrogenic; occurs in patients who get intra-articular injections.

SOURCE & TRANSMISSION:
- These bacteria are often normal flora of the **colon**.
- Transmission is mostly **nosocomial** via **urinary catheter**, via respiratory equipment, via IV lines or via IV injections. This occurs as an **opportunistic** infection in immunocompromised or otherwise debilitated patients.
- Horizontal transmission is common due to lack of hand washing.

VIRULENCE FACTORS:
- **Endotoxin**.
- **Multiple antibiotic resistance**.
- **Note:** pigmented strains may be less virulent than non-pigmented strains.

TREATMENT:
- **Ampicillin** for cystitis.
- **TMP-SMZ** for pyelonephritis, or for cystitis in penicillin allergy.
- **Amikacin** for resistant strains.

VACCINE & TOXOID:
None

HOST DEFENSE & IMMUNITY:
- In general, immune-competent people have no trouble fighting *S. marsescens*
- IgA, IgM, IgG **antibodies** to various cell surface components.
- **PMNs** respond in **acute** infections.
- **Macros** and **lymphocytes** respond in **chronic** infections.

LAB TESTS:
• Produces **red pigment**	
• Oxidase	Neg
• Lactose	Neg
• Indole	Neg
• Methyl Red	Neg
• **Voges-Proskauer**	**Pos**
• **Simmon's citrate**	**Pos**
• TSI (H_2S)	Neg
• Urease	+/-

Uropathogenic Escherichia coli

GRAM STAIN:
NEG

AEROBIC

EXTRACELLULAR

FEATURES:
- **Rods** : singly, pairs, chains.
- **Colonies:** gray, sometimes mucoid; on blood agar.

MOTILITY:
sometimes
Flagella

CAPSULE & GLYCOCALYX:
Sometimes **Capsule:**
Polysaccharide.

EXOTOXINS:
- **Hemolysins:** (disrupt blood cell membranes)
  - Some hemolysins disrupt RBCs to release iron which is required by *E. coli* for its own metabolic processes.
  - α-hemolysin: secreted; disrupts lymphocytes.
  - β-hemolysin: membrane-bound; inhibits PMNs.

ENDOTOXIN:
- **Lipopolysaccharide** (LPS): mediates septic shock.

CLINICAL:
- **UTI** (*E. coli* is #1 causative organism: 80%-95% of cases):
  - Upper (**pyelonephritis**) and lower (**cystitis**) urinary tract infections.
  - Symptoms:
    - **Pyelonephritis**: flank pain, **fever**, dysuria, ±cystitis symptoms.
    - **Cystitis**: dysuria, pyuria, ↑frequency, ↑urgency, ±hematuria.
  - Diagnosis: urine culture: >10^5 bacteria/ml.
  - Most **community** acquired infections are uncomplicated; present as **cystitis**; and are found in **women** due to **short urethra**.
  - Most **nosocomial** infections are complicated; present as **pyelonephritis**; and are found in **immunocompromised** patients due to in-dwelling catheters, urolithiasis, or other **obstruction**. Infections may progress to bacteremia or sepsis.
  - Infections may be **acute** or **chronic**.
- **Bacteremia and Sepsis** (*E. coli* is #1 causative nosocomial organism):
  - Often as a complication of pyelonephritis or iatrogenic from IV lines; may lead to **pneumonia** or **septic shock**; can be **fatal**.
- **Neonate Meningitis** (*E. coli* is #2 causative organism)
  - Symptoms: fever, lethargy, poor feeding. Seizures = poor prognosis.
  - Invades via mucus membranes, respiratory tract, and **sepsis**; often **fatal**.
  - Meningitis must be diagnosed via lumbar puncture:
    - CSF: ↑PMNs, ↓Glucose, Cloudy, Culture.
  - **Early onset** (age 0-5 days):
    Vertical transmission in utero; ascending, due to ruptured amnionic sac.
  - **Late onset** (age 5-90 days):
    Vertical transmission at time of delivery; or can be nosocomial.

SOURCE & TRANSMISSION:
- *E. coli* is often part of normal flora of the **colon**.
- Infection arises via **autoinoculation** (**fecal** contamination of the urethra, or **nosocomial** via urinary catheterization.
- Horizontal transmission is common due to lack of hand washing.
- **Vertically** transmitted either at birth or via ascension in utero.

VIRULENCE FACTORS:
- **Exotoxins.**
- **Endotoxin:** (O-antigens): provides antigenic variation.
  - Most infections are due to strains O-4, O-6, O-75.
- **Capsule:** (K-antigens): provides antigenic variation.
  - K-antigen-expressing strains are associated with **pyelonephritis**.
  - **K-1 strains** are associated with **meningitis** and **bacteremia**.
- **Flagella:** (H-antigens): provides antigenic variation as well as motility.
- **Pili:**(**P-Fimbria** in UTI; **S-Fimbria** in neonatal meningitis):
  - Mediates attachment to epithelial cells of the urinary tract.
- **Siderophores:** chelate host iron and enhance iron uptake into organism.
- *E. coli* has a great ability to resist opsonization by complement.

TREATMENT:
- **Ampicillin** for cystitis.
- **TMP-SMZ** for pyelonephritis, or for cystitis in penicillin allergy.
- **Ampicillin plus Gentamicin** for neonatal meningitis.

VACCINE & TOXOID:

None

HOST DEFENSE & IMMUNITY:
- IgA, IgM, IgG **antibodies** to various cell surface components.
- Host sequesters iron (required by *E. coli*) with blood transferrin and PMN lactoferrin.
- **PMNs** respond in **acute** infections.
- **Macros** and **lymphocytes** respond in **chronic** infections.

LAB TESTS:
● Oxidase	Neg
● **Lactose**	**Pos**
(Pink colonies on MacConkey)	
● **Indole**	**Pos**
● **Methyl Red**	**Pos**
● Voges-Proskauer	Neg
● Simmon's citrate	Neg
● TSI (H_2S)	Neg
● Urease	Neg

Chapter 8

GRAM NEGATIVE RODS Gastro-Intestinal Tract Related

STOMACH

Helicobacter pylori
       (Lumenal)
       Chronic gastritis
       Duodenal peptic ulcer
       Gastric peptic ulcer
       Gastric carcinoma

SMALL INTESTINES

Vibrio cholera
       (Lumenal)
       (Toxin)
       Cholera diarrhea

EnteroToxigenic Escherichia coli
       (Lumenal)
       (Toxin)
       Traveler's diarrhea

EnteroPathogenic Escherichia coli
(sometimes called EnteroAdherant E. coli)
       (Lumenal)
       Childhood diarrhea

EnteroAggregative Escherichia coli
       (Lumenal)
       Childhood diarrhea

SMALL AND LARGE INTESTINES

Campylobacter jejuni
       (Invasive)   (Zoonotic)
       Enterocolitis diarrhea
       Reiter syndrome

Yersinia enterocolitica
       (Invasive)   (Zoonotic)
       Enterocolitis diarrhea
       Sepsis
       Reiter syndrome

Salmonella enteritidis
Salmonella typhimurium
       (Invasive)   (Zoonotic)
       Enterocolitis
       Bacteremia
       Osteomyelitis
       Reiter syndrome

Salmonella typhi
Salmonella paratyphoid
       (Invasive)
       Enteric fever: Typhoid fever

Vibrio parahaemolyticus
       (Invasive)
       Food poisoning diarrhea

LARGE INTESTINES

EnteroHemorrhagic Escherichia coli
(O157:H7)
       (Lumenal)
       (Toxin)
       Hemorrhagic colitis
       Hemolytic-Uremic syndrome

Shigella spp
       (Invasive)
       (Toxin)
       Bacillary dysentery
       Hemolytic-Uremic syndrome
       Reiter syndrome

EnteroInvasive Escherichia coli
       (Invasive)
       Inflammatory dysentery

Helicobacter pylori

GRAM STAIN:
NEG

MICROAEROPHILIC

EXTRACELLULAR

FEATURES:
- Rods : **S-shape, comma shape.**
- Colonies: grow on selective media.

MOTILITY:
Amphitrichous Flagella:
"Cork-screw" movement.

CAPSULE & GLYCOCALYX:
None

EXOTOXINS:
None.

ENDOTOXIN:
- Lipopolysaccharide (LPS).

CLINICAL:
- **Chronic Gastritis (Type B)** (*H. pylori* is #1 causative organism):
  - Chronic infection follows acute infection.
  - *H. pylori* causes **superficial** mucosal inflammation of the **antrum** and **body** of the **stomach**; it is **non-invasive.**
  - Symptoms: this causes some nausea or upper abdominal discomfort, but, in many cases, the patient is **asymptomatic.**
  - 100% of chronic gastritis patients have *H. pylori* infection.
- **Duodenal Peptic Ulcer** (*H. pylori* is #1 causative organism):
  - Occurs in the **setting of** *H. pylori* **chronic gastritis.**
  - Symptoms: burning upper abdominal pain; occurs 1-3 hrs **after meals**; pain is worse at night but relieved by eating or use of antacids.
  - Diagnosis:
    - -Endoscopy with biopsy of gastric antrum.
    - -Serological tests helpful but not reliable to follow eradication.
    - -Breath test: *H. pylori* hydrolyzes carbon-labeled urea which can be detected in a sample of the patient's breath.
  - This ulceration is most often **chronic** and **recurrent**, and may lead to **complications** such as bleeding, anemia and perforation.
  - 90%-100% of duodenal peptic ulcer patients have *H. pylori* infection.
- **Gastric Peptic Ulcer** (*H. pylori* is #1 causative organism): similar to duodenal, except only 50%-80% of gastric peptic ulcers are associated with *H. pylori*.
- **Gastric Carcinoma:** occurs in the **setting of** *H. pylori* **chronic gastritis.**

SOURCE & TRANSMISSION:
- Human **GI tracts** are the only reservoirs for *H. pylori*.
- Horizontal transmission occurs via the **fecal-oral** route; especially in crowded living conditions.
- There is a direct relationship between **increased age** and increased likelihood of *H. pylori* infection in developed countries.

VIRULENCE FACTORS:
- **Endotoxin**: (O-antigens): provides antigenic variation.
- *H. pylori* has a great ability to **resist destruction by stomach acid.**
- **Flagella** with **corkscrew motility** enables movement into and within the protective mucus layer of the stomach.
- **Enzymes:**
  - **Urease** generates ammonium ions to buffer gastric acid; this enables survival within the hostile acidic environment.
  - **Mucinase** helps to break through the protective mucus layer.
- **Microaerophilism** enables survival within the mucus layer of stomach.
- **Adhesion factors:**
  - Mediate attachment to epithelial cells of the **stomach.**

TREATMENT:
- Combination of the following:
  - **Ranitidine** (H2 blocker)
  - plus **Bismuth salts** (Pepto Bismol)
  - plus **Amoxicillin**
  - plus **Metronidazole.**
- **Tetracycline** can be substituted for amoxicillin in penicillin allergy.
- Alternative combination:
  - Omeprazole (proton pump blocker)
  - plus Clarithromycin
  - plus Metronidazole.

VACCINE & TOXOID:

None

HOST DEFENSE & IMMUNITY:
- Strong **chronic inflammatory** response with Monos, Macros and Lymphos in the gastric mucosa (mostly the antrum).
- *H. pylori* remains in the gastric lumen; it is **non-invasive.**

LAB TESTS:
Oxidase	Pos
Catalase	Pos
TSI (H_2S)	Neg
Urease	Pos
Nitrate reduction	Neg
Hippurate hydrolysis	Neg
Cephalothin	Susceptible
Nalidixic acid	Resistant

Vibrio cholera

GRAM STAIN:
NEG

AEROBIC

EXTRACELLULAR

FEATURES:
- Rods : **S-shape, comma shape.**
- Colonies: grows on blood agar.

MOTILITY:
Polar
Monotrichous
Flagellum

CAPSULE & GLYCOCALYX:
None.

EXOTOXINS:
- **Enterotoxin:**
  - **LT** (Heat Labile Toxin) **Cholera Toxin:**
    Coded on **chromosome.**
    Functions in the **small intestines.**
    Activates stimulatory G-protein: (turns **on** the **on** signal)
    Five B-subunits:
    Bind to GM1 ganglioside of mucosal cell membranes; mediates entry of the A-unit.
    One A-subunit: causes addition of ADP-Ribose to G_s-protein:
    ↑**adenylate cyclase** , causes ↑**cAMP**;
    mucosal cells secrete Cl^- into lumen, water follows.

ENDOTOXIN:
- **Lipopolysaccharide** (LPS).

CLINICAL:
- **Cholera:**
  - *V. cholera* remains in **lumen** of **small intestines**, mostly the duodenum; it is **non-invasive.**
  - Symptoms: **painless**, voluminous and odorless **"rice-water" diarrhea** (the "rice" is mucus), **no fever.** The symptoms rapidly progress to include hypotension, dehydration, hypovolemia and shock. Can be **rapidly fatal** (hrs).
  - Diagnosis is made based on symptoms, history, and stool culture; treatment must be administered immediately.
  - Complications: electrolyte losses and imbalances, metabolic acidosis, hypoglycemia (especially in children), abortion (in pregnancy).
  - Infection requires a very **large infective dose (10^7 organisms)** because *V. cholera* is easily destroyed by stomach acid.

SOURCE & TRANSMISSION:
- Human **GI tract** is reservoir for *V. Cholera*
- *V. Cholera* may exist free-living in fresh water.
- Horizontal transmission occurs via **fecal-oral** route, especially from drinking **contaminated water.**
- **Epidemics** can occur anywhere.

VIRULENCE FACTORS:
- **Exotoxin.**
- **Endotoxin:** (O-antigens): provides antigenic variation.
  - **O1 strains** can cause epidemics
  - **Non-O1 strains** can cause sporadic infections but not epidemics.
- **Flagellum** (H-antigens) and curved shape:
  - Provides strong motility; enables penetration into mucus layer.
  - Provides antigenic variation .
- **Adhesion factors:**
  - Mediate attachment to epithelial cells of the **small intestines.**

TREATMENT:
- Immediate and continuous oral or IV **replacement of fluids and electrolytes** is absolutely essential.
- A solution of table salt plus cooked rice together in water can substitute as an oral home-treatment alternative.
- **Tetracycline** to speed-up recovery.
- **Prevention:** good hygiene and good waste water treatment.

VACCINE & TOXOID:
Ineffective vaccine:
killed bacteria

HOST DEFENSE & IMMUNITY:
- **Stomach acid** kills *V. cholera*, therefore, only a very large dose can cause infection.
- **Sectreted IgA**, and exudate IgG antibodies to various components and to cholera toxin.
- Previous infection confers long lasting type-specific immunity.
- *V. cholera* remains in the intestinal lumen; it is **non-invasive.**
- *V. cholera* can not colonize the large intestines because it can not compete with the commensal anaerobic bacteria there.

LAB TESTS:
- **Oxidase**   Pos
- **Lactose**   Pos
  (Pink colonies on MacConkey)
- **Indole**   Pos
- **Methyl Red**   Pos
- Urease   Neg
- **TCBS agar**   yellow colonies
      (ferments sucrose)
- 7% NaCl   No growth
- Alkaline   Growth

EnteroToxigenic Escherichia coli

GRAM STAIN:
NEG

AEROBIC

EXTRACELLULAR

FEATURES:
- **Rods** : singly, pairs, chains.
- **Colonies**: gray, sometimes mucoid; on blood agar.

MOTILITY:
sometimes
Flagella

CAPSULE & GLYCOCALYX:
Sometimes **Capsule**:
Polysaccharide.

EXOTOXINS:
- **Enterotoxins:** (coded on plasmids):
  - **LT** (Heat Labile Toxin) "**Cholera-Like Toxin:**"
    Functions in the **small intestines.**
    Activates stimulatory G-protein: (turns on the on signal)
    Five B-subunits:
    Bind to GM1 ganglioside of mucosal cell membranes; mediates entry of the A-unit.
    One A-subunit: causes addition of ADP-Ribose to G_s-protein:
    ↑**adenylate cyclase** , causes ↑**cAMP**;
    mucosal cells secrete Cl⁻ into lumen, water follows.
  - **ST** (Heat stable Toxin):
    Activates **guanylate cyclase**; ↑cGMP;
    blocks ion transport from lumen into cells;
    so water then flows into lumen.

ENDOTOXIN:
- **Lipopolysaccharide** (LPS).

CLINICAL:
- **T**raveler's **Diarrhea:** (Enteritis):
  - ETEC remains in **lumen** of **small intestines**, it is **non-invasive.**
  - Symptoms: mild or explosive **watery diarrhea**, nausea, vomiting.
    Symptoms arise within 2-3 days of ingestion of the bacteria.
    Symptoms last about 4 days.
  - Infection occurs mostly in **adults** from industrialized countries who **travel** to the tropics (Mexico, Africa, Asia).

SOURCE & TRANSMISSION:
- **ETEC** may be part of normal intestinal flora of people in the endemic area.
- Horizontal transmission occurs via **fecal-oral** route when travelers ingest fecal-contaminated food or water, especially raw vegetables.

VIRULENCE FACTORS:
- **Exotoxins**.
- **Endotoxin**: (O-antigens): provides antigenic variation.
- **Capsule**: (K-antigens): provides antigenic variation.
- **Flagella**: (H-antigens): provides antigenic variation as well as motility.
- **Pili**: (Fimbria): also known as **Colonization factor Antigen (CFA)**:
  - Coded on a plasmid.
  - Provides antigenic variation.
  - Mediates attachment to epithelial cells of the **small intestines.**

TREATMENT:
- Infection is most often **self-limited.**
- **Fluid and electrolyte replacement** is necessary.
- Prophylaxis is not recommended, but **prevention** can be achieved by eating only cooked foods and drinking only bottled water while traveling.

VACCINE & TOXOID:

None

HOST DEFENSE & IMMUNITY:
- Secreted **IgA antibodies** to fimbriae.
- Previous infection confers long lasting type-specific immunity.
- ETEC remains in the intestinal lumen; it is **non-invasive.**

LAB TESTS:

● Oxidase	Neg
● **Lactose**	**Pos**
(Pink colonies on MacConkey)	
● **Indole**	**Pos**
● **Methyl Red**	**Pos**
● Voges-Proskauer	Neg
● Simmon's citrate	Neg
● TSI (H_2S)	Neg
● Urease	Neg

EnteroPathogenic Escherichia coli

GRAM STAIN:
NEG

AEROBIC

EXTRACELLULAR

FEATURES:
- **Rods** : singly, pairs, chains.
- **Colonies:** gray, sometimes mucoid; on blood agar.

MOTILITY:
sometimes
Flagella

CAPSULE & GLYCOCALYX:
Sometimes **Capsule**:
Polysaccharide.

EXOTOXINS:
- Enterotoxin.

ENDOTOXIN:
- **Lipopolysaccharide** (LPS).

CLINICAL:
- **Childhood Diarrhea:** (Enteritis):
  - **EPEC** remains in **lumen** of **small intestines**. It is **non-invasive**, but can **disrupt the mucus layer**, and **destroy microvilli**.
  - Symptoms: diarrhea, nausea, vomiting, and **mucus** in the stools.
  - Infection occurs mostly in **young children**, especially in day-care centers or nursery schools; mostly in developing countries.
- **Note:** EPEC strains are sometimes called "Enteroadherent *E. coli*" or EAEC

SOURCE & TRANSMISSION:
- **EPEC** may be part of normal intestinal flora of some people.
- Horizontal transmission occurs via **fecal-oral** route from child to child, when children are living, eating or playing together.
- Transmission also occurs via **fecal-oral** route from drinking contaminated water.

VIRULENCE FACTORS:
- **Exotoxin**.
- **Endotoxin**: (O-antigens): provides antigenic variation.
- **Capsule**: (K-antigens): provides antigenic variation.
- **Flagella**: (H-antigens): provides antigenic variation as well as motility.
- **Pili**: (Fimbria): also known as EPEC **Adhesion Factor**:
  - Two kinds: one coded on a plasmid, and one on a chromosome (*eae* gene).
  - Provides antigenic variation.
  - Mediates **focal attachment** to specific epithelial cells of the **small intestines**.

TREATMENT:
- Infection is most often **self-limited.**
- **Fluid and electrolyte replacement** is necessary.

VACCINE & TOXOID:

None

HOST DEFENSE & IMMUNITY:
- Secreted **IgA antibodies** to fimbriae.
- Previous infection confers long lasting type-specific immunity.
- **EPEC** remains in the intestinal lumen; it is **non-invasive**.

LAB TESTS:	
●Oxidase	Neg
●**Lactose**	**Pos**
(Pink colonies on MacConkey)	
●**Indole**	**Pos**
●**Methyl Red**	**Pos**
●Voges-Proskauer	Neg
●Simmon's citrate	Neg
●TSI (H$_2$S)	Neg
●Urease	Neg

EnteroAggregative Escherichia coli

GRAM STAIN:
NEG

AEROBIC

EXTRACELLULAR

FEATURES:
- **Rods** : singly, pairs, chains.
- **Colonies**: gray, sometimes mucoid; on blood agar.

MOTILITY:
sometimes
Flagella

CAPSULE & GLYCOCALYX:
Sometimes **Capsule**:
Polysaccharide.

EXOTOXINS:
- Enterotoxin.

ENDOTOXIN:
- **Lipopolysaccharide (LPS)**.

CLINICAL:
- **Childhood Diarrhea:** (Enteritis):
  - ▪EAggEC remains in **lumen** of **small intestines**. It is **non-invasive**, but it can **disrupt the mucus layer**, and **destroy microvilli**.
  - ▪They differ from EPEC because of their ability to aggressively, and specifically attach to certain mucosal cells.
  - ▪Symptoms: **persistent diarrhea**, nausea, vomiting. Mucus and sometimes **blood** can be found in the stool.
  - ▪Infection occurs mostly in **young children**, especially in day-care centers or nursery schools; mostly in developing countries.

SOURCE & TRANSMISSION:
- **EAggEC** may be part of normal intestinal flora of some people.
- Horizontal transmission occurs via **fecal-oral** route from child to child, when children are living, eating or playing together.
- Transmission also occurs via **fecal-oral** route from drinking contaminated water.

VIRULENCE FACTORS:
- **Exotoxin**.
- **Endotoxin**: (O-antigens): provides antigenic variation.
- **Capsule**: (K-antigens): provides antigenic variation.
- **Flagella**: (H-antigens): provides antigenic variation as well as motility.
- **Pili**: (Fimbria):
  - ▪Coded on a **plasmid**.
  - ▪Provides antigenic variation.
  - ▪Mediates **aggressive attachment** to **specific epithelial cells** of the **small intestines**.

TREATMENT:
- Infection is most often **self-limited**.
- **Fluid and electrolyte replacement** is necessary.

VACCINE & TOXOID:

None

HOST DEFENSE & IMMUNITY:
- Secreted **IgA antibodies** to fimbriae.
- Previous infection confers long lasting type-specific immunity.
- **EaggEC** remains in the intestinal lumen; it is **non-invasive**.

LAB TESTS:
●Oxidase	Neg
●**Lactose**	**Pos**
(Pink colonies on MacConkey)	
●**Indole**	**Pos**
●**Methyl Red**	**Pos**
●Voges-Proskauer	Neg
●Simmon's citrate	Neg
●TSI (H$_2$S)	Neg
●Urease	Neg

Campylobacter jejuni

GRAM STAIN:
NEG

Zoonotic

MICROAEROPHILIC

EXTRACELLULAR

FEATURES:
- Rods : **S-shape, comma shape**.
pairs resemble "seagulls"
- Colonies: grow slowly on selective media.

MOTILITY:
Monotrichous
Flagellum
Darting movement

CAPSULE & GLYCOCALYX:
None.

EXOTOXINS:
Enterotoxin and cytotoxin produced, but without significance.

ENDOTOXIN:
- **Lipopolysaccharide** (LPS).

CLINICAL:
- **Enterocolitis:**
  - *C. jejuni* **invades** the mucosal cells of the **jejunum, ileum** and **large intestines**. *C. jejuni* thrives in bile secretions. The invasion does **not** progress to become a systemic invasion.
  - Symptoms: **fever**, nausea, abdominal pain and **watery diarrhea** or **bloody diarrhea** with **inflammation** and **pus in stool**. Symptoms arise within 48 hrs of ingesting the bacteria. Symptoms last about 5 days.
  - Symptoms can **mimic appendicitis**.
  - Infections by *C. jejuni* are **very common**, especially in **children** and **young adults**.
- Post-Campylobacter **Reiter Syndrome**:
  - Arthritic disease associated with HLA-B27 genotype.

SOURCE & TRANSMISSION:
- **Animals** are reservoirs for *C. Jejuni*, so **Zoonotic transmission** occurs via **contact** with animals: **dogs**, cats, farm animals, and fowl, especially **chicken** and **turkey**.
- Transmission also occurs via ingesting **food products** from the infected animals due to contamination during slaughtering; via **raw milk**; or by ingesting **water** contaminated by animal **feces** (e.g. while backpacking).
- Horizontal transmission occurs via **fecal-oral** route from **child to child**, when children are living, eating or playing together.

VIRULENCE FACTORS:
- **Endotoxin**: (O-antigens): provides antigenic variation.
- **Flagella**: (H-antigens):
  - Provides antigenic variation.
  - Flagella antigen undergoes **variation** by **gene rearrangement**.
  - Provides characteristic **darting motility**.
- *C. jejuni* thrives in human bile.

TREATMENT:
- Infection is most often **self-limited.**
- **Fluid and electrolyte replacement** is necessary.
- **Erythromycin** in severe cases.
- **Prevention:** good hygiene, especially after handling animals. And avoidance of contaminated water especially when back-packing.

Cipro

VACCINE & TOXOID:
None

HOST DEFENSE & IMMUNITY:
- Strong **acute inflammatory** response with PMNs.
- **T-Cell** mediated immunity is important.
- Secreted **IgA** and **IgG** exudate antibodies to various bacterial components.
- Previous infection confers long lasting immunity.

LAB TESTS:
- **Oxidase**   **Pos**
- **Catalase**   **Pos**
- Urease   Neg
- Nitrate reduction   Neg
- **Hippurate hydrolysis   Pos**
- **Cephalothin   Resistant**
- Nalidixic acid   Susceptible

Yersinia enterocolitica

GRAM STAIN:
NEG

Zoonotic

AEROBIC

EXTRACELLULAR

FEATURES:
- **Rods** : coccobacilli.
- Colonies: grow on blood agar.

MOTILITY:
Flagellum
but **not motile**
in host.

CAPSULE & GLYCOCALYX:
Unknown

EXOTOXINS:
Enterotoxin is produced but without significance.

ENDOTOXIN:
- **Lipopolysaccharide** (LPS).

CLINICAL:
- **Enterocolitis:**
  - *Y. enterocolitica* **invades** the mucosal cells of the **ileum** and **large intestines**. The invasion may progress to the **Peyer's patches**.
  - Symptoms: **fever**, nausea, abdominal pain and **watery diarrhea** or **bloody diarrhea** with **inflammation** and **pus in stool**. Perforation of the ileum may occur in severe cases. Symptoms arise within 1 week of ingesting the bacteria. Symptoms last about 2 weeks.
  - Symptoms can **mimic appendicitis**.
  - Infection requires a very **large infective dose (10^9 organisms)** because *Y. enterocolitica* are easily destroyed by stomach acid.
  - *Y. enterocolitica*, although *uncommon*, infect mostly **children**.
- **Bacteremia** and **Sepsis:**
  - Mostly in **iron-overload** patients due to **multiple blood transfusions**.
  - Very often **fatal**.
- **Post-Yersinia Reiter Syndrome:**
  - Arthritic disease associated with HLA-B27 genotype.

SOURCE & TRANSMISSION:
- **Animals** are reservoirs for *Y. enterocolitica*, so **Zoonotic transmission** occurs via **contact** with animals: **dogs**, cats, farm animals and rodents, especially in **Scandinavia.**
- Transmission also occurs via ingesting **food products** from the infected animals due to contamination during slaughtering; via **raw milk**; via cold meat; or by ingesting **water** contaminated by animal **feces**.

VIRULENCE FACTORS:
- **Endotoxin**: (O-antigens): provides antigenic variation.
- **Flagella**: (H-antigens):
  - Provides antigenic variation.
  - Motility is observed in culture at 25°C but not in host at 37°C.
- **Special Requirements:**
  - Iron (they do not have a siderophore and require the presence of other organisms to supply them with iron.)
  - Calcium
- Ability to resist serum complement (coded on plasmid).
- Ability to grow in **cold conditions** such as refrigeration.

TREATMENT:
- Infection is most often **self-limited.**
- **Fluid and electrolyte replacement** is necessary.
- **Gentamicin** in **sepsis** cases.
- **Prevention:** good hygiene, especially after handling animals. Incubation of blood in blood banks before storage.

VACCINE & TOXOID:
None

HOST DEFENSE & IMMUNITY:
- Strong **acute inflammatory** response with PMNs.
- Secreted **IgA** and **IgG** exudate antibodies to various bacterial components.
- Previous infection confers long lasting immunity.
- Complement is ineffective.

LAB TESTS:

Oxidase	Neg
Catalase	**Pos**
Lactose	Neg
Indole	+/-
Methyl Red	**Pos**
Voges-Proskauer	Neg
Simmon's citrate	+/-
TSI (H2S)	Neg
Urease	**Pos**

Salmonella enteritidis
Salmonella typhimurium

GRAM STAIN:
NEG

"Non-Typhoidal *Salmonella*"

Zoonotic

AEROBIC

INTRACELLULAR

FEATURES:
- **Rods** : singly, pairs, chains.
- Colonies: gray; on blood agar.

MOTILITY:
Flagella

CAPSULE & GLYCOCALYX:
Capsule:
Polysaccharide.

EXOTOXINS:
None.

_____

ENDOTOXIN:
- **Lipopolysaccharide** (LPS).

CLINICAL:
- **Enterocolitis:**
  - *S. enteriditis* and *S. Typhimurium* **invade** the mucosal cells of the **ileum** and **large intestines**. The invasion may progress to become a **systemic invasion**.
  - Symptoms: **fever**, nausea, vomiting and **watery diarrhea** with **inflammation** and **pus in stool**.
    Symptoms arise within 48 hrs of ingesting the bacteria.
    Symptoms last about 7 days but the *Salmonella* organisms may be carried in the stool for more than a month.
  - Symptoms can **mimic appendicitis**.
  - Infection requires a very **large infective dose** (10^5 **organisms**) because *Salmonella* are easily destroyed by stomach acid.
- **Bacteremia** (results from spread of the enteric infection to the blood stream):
  - May lead to infections elsewhere: arterial infections, endocarditis, billiary tract infections, septic arthritis, and others.
  - Recurrent *Salmonella* bacteremia occurs in **AIDS** patients.
- **Osteomyelitis:** *Salmonella* bone infection arises from hematogenous spread; especially in children with **sickle cell disease**.
- Post-Salmonellosis **Reiter Syndrome**:
  - Arthritic disease associated with HLA-B27 genotype.

SOURCE & TRANSMISSION:
- **Animals** are **zoonotic** reservoirs for non-typhoidal *Salmonella*, so food products such as **eggs**, **milk**, and **chicken** are sources.
- Transmission occurs via ingestion of the **infected food**.
- **Horizontal transmission** may occur via **fecal-oral** route when children are living, eating, playing together.
- **Zoonotic transmission** may occur via contact with animals.
- **Chronic carrier** status is possible.

VIRULENCE FACTORS:
- **Endotoxin**: (O-antigens): provides antigenic variation.
- **Capsule**: (K-antigens): provides antigenic variation.
- **Flagella**: (H-antigens): provides antigenic variation as well as motility.
- *Salmonella* have the ability to **survive within Macros** (but not PMNs).
- **Invasion factor:**
  - Coded on a chromosome.
  - Mediates **invasion of** mucus layer and invasion of epithelial cells of the ileum and small intestine.
- **Multiple Drug Resistance Enzymes** (coded on plasmid):
  - **β-Lactamase**: for penicillin resistance.
  - **Acetlytransferase** to break down chloramphenicol.

TREATMENT:
- Infection is most often **self-limited**.
- **Fluid and electrolyte replacement** is necessary.
- **Ciprofloxacin** or **TMP-SMZ** for systemic infections.
- **Ciprofloxacin** for chronic carriers.
- **Prevention:**
  Avoid raw eggs (Caesar salads)
  Avoid under-cooked chicken.
  Wash your hands always before eating.
  Avoid antacids.

VACCINE & TOXOID:

None

HOST DEFENSE & IMMUNITY:
- Strong **acute inflammatory** response with PMNs.
- **T-Cell** mediated immunity is important.
- Secreted **IgA** and exudate IgG antibodies to various bacterial components.
- **Stomach acid** kills *Salmonella* therefore, only a very large dose can cause infection.

LAB TESTS:

Oxidase	Neg
Lactose	Neg
Indole	Neg
Methyl Red	**Pos**
Voges-Proskauer	Neg
Simmon's citrate	+/-
TSI (H$_2$S)	**Pos**
Urease	Neg

Salmonella typhi
Salmonella paratyphi

GRAM STAIN:
NEG

"Typhoidal *Salmonella*"

AEROBIC

INTRACELLULAR

FEATURES:
- **Rods** : singly, pairs, chains.
- Colonies: gray; on blood agar.

MOTILITY:
Flagella

CAPSULE & GLYCOCALYX:
Capsule:
Polysaccharide.

EXOTOXINS:
None.

ENDOTOXIN:
- **Lipopolysaccharide (LPS).**

CLINICAL:
- **Enteric Fever** (Typhoid Fever and Paratyphoid Fever):
  - *S. typhi* and *S. paratyphi* **invade** the **Peyer's Patches** of the **ileum** and **large intestines**. The invasion progresses via **thoracic duct** to become a **systemic invasion**.
  - Symptoms: **fever**, enterocolitis with **diarrhea** and abdominal pain, hepatosplenomegaly, **bradycardia**, and **rose spots on trunk**. **Late symptoms** (4 wks): intestinal hemorrhage and delirium. Symptoms arise within 7+ days of ingesting the bacteria. Symptoms last about 1 month if untreated, or 1 week if treated. Enteric Fever can be **fatal** or relapsing.
  - Infection requires a very **large infective dose (10^5 organisms)** because *Salmonella* are easily destroyed by stomach acid.
- **Abortion:**
  Most pregnancies will end in abortion during Enteric fever.
- **Bacteremia**

SOURCE & TRANSMISSION:
- **Human GI tract** is reservoir for *S. typhi* and *S. paratyphi*. Especially S.E. Asia, Africa, and Latin America.
- **Horizontal** transmission occurs via **fecal-oral** route, especially from drinking contaminated water.
- **Chronic carrier** status is possible.

VIRULENCE FACTORS:
- **Endotoxin**: (O-antigens): provides antigenic variation.
- **Capsule: Vi Antigen**: aids in resistance to antibodies and complement.
- **Flagella**: (H-antigens):
  - Provides antigenic variation as well as motility.
  - Flagella antigen undergoes variation by **gene rearrangement**.
- *Salmonella* have the ability to **survive within Macros** (but not PMNs).
- **Invasion factor:**
  - Coded on a chromosome.
  - Mediates **invasion of** mucus layer and invasion of epithelial cells of the ileum and small intestine.
- **Multiple Drug Resistance Enzymes** (coded on plasmid):
  - **β-Lactamase**: for penicillin resistance.
  - **Acetlytransferase** to break down chloramphenicol.

TREATMENT:
- **Ciprofloxacin** or **TMP-SMZ** for systemic infections.
- **Ciprofloxacin** for chronic carriers.
- **Prevention:**
  Observe good hygiene while traveling. Avoid antacids.
  β-lactames

VACCINE & TOXOID:
Ineffective vaccine:
killed bacteria

HOST DEFENSE & IMMUNITY:
- Strong **acute inflammatory** response with PMNs: resultant **Acute Leukopenia**.
- **T-Cell** mediated immunity is important.
- Secreted **IgA** and exudate **IgG** antibodies to various bacterial components.
- Previous infection confers long lasting type-specific **immunity**.
- **Stomach acid** kills *Salmonella* therefore, only a very large dose can cause infection.

LAB TESTS:

Oxidase	Neg
Lactose	Neg
Indole	Neg
Methyl Red	**Pos**
Voges-Proskauer	Neg
Simmon's citrate	+/-
TSI (H$_2$S)	**Pos**
Urease	Neg

Vibrio parahaemolyticus

GRAM STAIN:
NEG

AEROBIC

EXTRACELLULAR

FEATURES:
- Rods : **S-shape, comma shape.**
- Colonies: green;
grows on TCBS agar.

MOTILITY:
Polar

Monotrichous

Flagellum

CAPSULE & GLYCOCALYX:
None.

EXOTOXINS:
- **Enterotoxin:**
      An agent of food poisoning.
- **Cytotoxin.**

ENDOTOXIN:
- **Lipopolysaccharide** (LPS).

CLINICAL:
- **Food Poisoning:**
    - **Enterotoxin**, preformed when *V. parahaemolyticus* colonizes food, is toxic to the mucosal cells of the **small intestines.**
    - *V. parahaemolyticus* **invade** the mucosal cells of the **large intestine,** but invasion does **not** progress to become systemic.
    - Symptoms: abdominal pain with **explosive watery diarrhea**.
    - Symptoms arise within 24 hrs of **ingestion of contaminated food.** Symptoms are self-limited and last about 3 days.
    - Infection requires a very **large infective dose.**

SOURCE & TRANSMISSION:
- *V. parahaemolyticus* exists **free-living** in **salt water.**
- Disease arises from ingesting **raw or under-cooked seafood;** or from ingesting food contaminated be **sea water.**

VIRULENCE FACTORS:
- **Exotoxin.**
- **Endotoxin**: (O-antigens): provides antigenic variation.
- **Flagellum** and curved shape:
    - Provides strong motility; enables penetration into mucus layer.
    - Provides antigenic variation (H-antigens).
- **Halophilic:**
      Can thrive in **salt water** or on salt media.

TREATMENT:
- Infection is most often **self-limited.**
- **Fluid and electrolyte replacement** is necessary.
- **Prevention:** cook all seafood well.

VACCINE & TOXOID:

None.

HOST DEFENSE & IMMUNITY:
- Strong **acute inflammatory** response in reaction to enterotoxin.
- Secreted **IgA** and exudate IgG antibodies to various bacterial components.
- **Stomach acid** kills *V. parahaemolyticus* therefore, only a very large dose can cause infection.

LAB TESTS:
- **Oxidase**   Pos
- **Lactose**   Pos
(Pink colonies on MacConkey)
- **Indole**   Pos
- **Methyl Red**   Pos
- Urease   Neg
- **TCBS** agar   green colonies
(does not ferment sucrose)
- **7% NaCl**   **Growth**
- Alkaline   Growth

EnteroHemorrhagic Escherichia coli

GRAM STAIN:
NEG

Strain: "O157:H7"

AEROBIC

EXTRACELLULAR

FEATURES:
- Rods : singly, pairs, chains.
- Colonies: gray, sometimes mucoid; on blood agar.

MOTILITY:
sometimes
Flagella

CAPSULE & GLYCOCALYX:
Sometimes **Capsule**:
Polysaccharide.

EXOTOXINS:
- **Enterotoxins:** (coded by lysogeny from a **temperate bacteriophage**)
  - **Shiga-like Toxin I (SLT I):**
    Functions in the **large intestines**.
    Five B-subunits:
    Bind to glycoproteins of mucosal cell membranes; mediates entry of the A-unit.
    One A-subunit:
    Inactivates the 28s rRNA subunit within the 60s subunit of host mucosal cells to **stop protein synthesis**.
    This **kills mucosal cells** to cause bloody stools.
    This also prevents nutrient absorption.
  - **Shiga-like Toxin II (SLT II):**
    Function is similar to SLT I.
  - **Note**: these toxins were formerly called Vero Toxins due to their toxicity to the cells of Vero monkeys.

ENDOTOXIN:
- **Lipopolysaccharide** (LPS).

CLINICAL:
- **Hemorrhagic Colitis (non-inflammatory dysentery):**
  - **EHEC** remains in **lumen** of **large intestines**. It is **non-invasive**, but its toxins can destroy mucosal cells.
  - Symptoms: nausea with watery diarrhea that progresses to **bloody diarrhea** with **no fever** and **no inflammation**.
  - Infection is mostly found in **children**, but can be **fatal** in the **elderly**.
- **Hemolytic-Uremic Syndrome:**
  - Symptoms: acute renal failure, hemolytic anemia, thrombocytopenia.
  - Infection occurs mostly in children.
- Note: most EHEC infections are caused by one strain: O157:H7.

SOURCE & TRANSMISSION:
- Human **GI tract** is reservoir for EHEC.
- Horizontal transmission occurs via **fecal-oral** route, especially from drinking contaminated water.
- Transmission has been known to occur via **fecal-oral** route from eating **undercooked hamburger** in fast-food restaurants.

VIRULENCE FACTORS:
- **Exotoxins**.
- **Endotoxin**: (O-antigens): provides antigenic variation.
- **Capsule**: (K-antigens): provides antigenic variation.
- **Flagella**: (H-antigens): provides antigenic variation as well as motility.
- **Pili**: (Fimbria):
  - Coded on a plasmid.
  - Provides antigenic variation.
  - Mediates attachment to epithelial cells of the **large intestines**.

TREATMENT:
- Infection is most often **self-limited.**
- **Fluid and electrolyte replacement** is necessary.

VACCINE & TOXOID:
None

HOST DEFENSE & IMMUNITY:
- Note the **lack of inflammation**.
- Secreted IgA and exudate IgG antibodies to various bacterial components.
- Previous infection confers long lasting type-specific immunity.
- EHEC remains in the intestinal lumen; it is **non-invasive**.

LAB TESTS:
- Oxidase — Neg
- **Lactose** — **Pos**
(Pink colonies on MacConkey)
- **Sorbitol** — **Neg**
(Colorless on Sorbitol-ManConkey)
- **Indole** — **Pos**
- **Methyl Red** — **Pos**
- Voges-Proskauer — Neg
- Simmon's citrate — Neg
- TSI (H_2S) — Neg
- Urease — Neg

Shigella spp

Shigella dysenteriae (group A)
Shigella flexneri (group B)
Shigella boydii (group C)
Shigella sonnei (group D)

GRAM STAIN:
NEG

AEROBIC

INTRACELLULAR

FEATURES:
- **Rods** : singly or pairs.
- Colonies: colorless
  on EMB agar.

MOTILITY:
None.

CAPSULE & GLYCOCALYX:
None.

EXOTOXINS:
- **Enterotoxin:**
  - **ShigaToxin:**
    Functions in the **large intestines**.
    Five B-subunits:
      Bind to glycoproteins of mucosal cell membranes;
      mediates entry of the A-unit.
    One A-subunit:
      Inactivates the 28s rRNA subunit within the 60s subunit
      of host mucosal cells to **stop protein synthesis**.
      This **kills mucosal cells** to cause bloody stools.
      This also prevents nutrient absorption.

ENDOTOXIN:
- **Lipopolysaccharide** (LPS).

CLINICAL:
- **Bacillary Dysentery** (Shigellosis):
  - *Shigella* **invade** the mucosal cells of the **large intestine**, but the
    invasion does **not** progress to become a systemic invasion.
  - Symptoms: fever and nausea with watery diarrhea progresses to
    bloody diarrhea with **inflammation** and **pus in stool**.
  - Symptoms arise within 1-3 days of infection as the bacteria descend
    through the small intestines to settle in the large intestines.
    Symptoms last about 7 days.
  - Infection requires a very **small infective dose**:
    as few as **50-300 organisms** can cause disease.
  - Infection occurs mostly in **young children**, especially in day-care
    centers or nursery schools; in the USA and other countries.
    Infections can be **fatal**, especially in elderly or in epidemics.
  - **Note**: currently, *S. sonnei* is the most prevalent agent of Shigellosis;
    however, the dominant species changes from generation to generation.
- **Hemolytic-Uremic Syndrome:**
  - Symptoms: acute renal failure, hemolytic anemia, thrombocytopenia.
  - Infection is mostly found in children.
- Post-Shigellosis **Reiter Syndrome**:
  - Arthritic disease associated with HLA-B27 genotype.

SOURCE & TRANSMISSION:
- **Human GI tract** is reservoir for *Shigella*.
- Horizontal transmission occurs via **fecal-oral** route from **child
  to child**, when children are living, eating or playing together.
- Transmission is common among **homosexual men**.
- **Bacillary dysentery** (Shigellosis) is **extremely contagious.**
- **Epidemics** can occur especially among troops during war.

VIRULENCE FACTORS:
- **Endotoxin**: (O-antigens): provides antigenic variation.
- *Shigella* have a great ability to **resist destruction by stomach acid**;
  this enables them to cause infection with only a few organisms.
- **Invasion factor** (similar to EIEC):
  - Coded on a plasmid.
  - Mediates **invasion and destruction** of colonic epithelium.
- Few organisms are necessary for infection.

TREATMENT:
- **TMP-SMZ** in serious cases or during
  epidemics **to stop transmission**. It has
  little effect on symptoms.
- Infection is most often **self-limited**.
- **Fluid and electrolyte replacement** is
  necessary.

VACCINE & TOXOID:

None.

HOST DEFENSE & IMMUNITY:
- Strong **acute inflammatory** response
  with PMNs.
- Secreted **IgA** and exudate IgG antibodies
  to various bacterial components.
- Previous infection confers long lasting
  type-specific immunity.
- *Shigella* invade only the intestinal mucosa;
  they do not progress to systemic infection.

LAB TESTS:
Oxidase	Neg
Lactose	Neg
Indole	+/-
Methyl Red	**Pos**
Voges-Proskauer	Neg
Simmon's citrate	Neg
TSI (H$_2$S)	Neg
Urease	Neg
Sereny test	**Pos**

Enteroinvasive Escherichia coli

GRAM STAIN:
NEG

AEROBIC

EXTRACELLULAR

FEATURES:
- **Rods** : singly, pairs, chains.
- Colonies: gray, sometimes mucoid; on blood agar.

MOTILITY:
sometimes
Flagella

CAPSULE & GLYCOCALYX:
Sometimes **Capsule**:
Polysaccharide.

EXOTOXINS:
None.

ENDOTOXIN:
- **Lipopolysaccharide** (LPS).

CLINICAL:
- **Enterocolitis** and **Inflammatory Dysentery:**
  - **EIEC invades** the mucosal cells of the **large intestine**, but invasion does **not** progress to become a systemic invasion.
  - Symptoms: fever and nausea with watery diarrhea progresses to **bloody diarrhea** with **inflammation** and **pus in stool**.
  - Note: these are shigella-like symptoms. Do not confuse EIEC with EHEC which produces a shigella-like toxin.
  - Infection caused by EIEC is **rare**, especially in the USA.

SOURCE & TRANSMISSION:
- Human **GI tract** is reservoir for EIEC.
- Horizontal transmission occurs via **fecal-oral** route, especially from drinking contaminated water.

VIRULENCE FACTORS:
- **Endotoxin**: (O-antigens): provides antigenic variation.
- **Capsule**: (K-antigens): provides antigenic variation.
- **Flagella**: (H-antigens): provides antigenic variation as well as motility.
- **Pili**: (Fimbria):
  - Coded on a plasmid.
  - Provides antigenic variation.
  - Mediates attachment to epithelial cells of the **large intestines**.
- **Invasion factor** (similar to *Shigella*):
  - Coded on a plasmid.
  - Mediates **invasion and destruction** of **colonic epithelium**.

TREATMENT:
- Infection is most often **self-limited.**
- **Fluid and electrolyte replacement** is necessary.

VACCINE & TOXOID:

None

HOST DEFENSE & IMMUNITY:
- Strong **acute inflammatory** response with **PMNs**.
- Secreted **IgA** and exudate IgG antibodies to various bacterial components.
- Previous infection confers long lasting type-specific immunity.
- **EIEC** invades only the intestinal mucosa; it does not progress to systemic infection.

LAB TESTS:
Oxidase	Neg
Lactose	**Pos**
(Pink colonies on MacConkey)	
Indole	**Pos**
Methyl Red	**Pos**
Voges-Proskauer	Neg
Simmon's citrate	Neg
TSI (H$_2$S)	Neg
Urease	Neg

Chapter 9

ZOONOTIC BACTERIA

ZOONOTIC TRANSMISSION:

Direct Contact.

Bites or Scratches.

Ingestion of animal food products.

Inhalation of animal bodily fluids.

Subsequent Horizontal or Vertical transmission is possible in some cases.

Vector transmission is possible in some cases.

MISCELLANEOUS

Bacillus anthracis
   Cutaneous Anthrax
   Respiratory Anthrax

Listeria monocytogenes
   (some **Vertical** transmission)
(see Gram Positive Rod chapter).

Mycobacterium bovis
   (some **Horizontal** transmission)
(see Gram Positive Rods:
   Acid-Fast Chapter)

Leptospira interrogans
(see Spirochete chapter)

Chlamydia psittaci
(see Chlamydia chapter)

ENTERIC-RELATED

Campylobacter jejuni
   (some **Horizontal** transmission)
(see Gram Negative Rods
Gastro-Intestinal Tract Chapter)

Yersinia enterocolitica
   (some **Horizontal** transmission)
(see Gram Negative Rods:
Gastro-Intestinal Tract Chapter)

Salmonella enteritidis

Salmonella typhimurium
   (some **Horizontal** transmission)
(see Gram Negative Rods:
Gastro-Intestinal Tract Chapter)

FEVER-RELATED

Brucella spp
   Brucellosis enteric fever
   Undulant fever

Coxiella burnetii
   (some **Vector** transmission)
   Q Fever acute febrile illness
   Q Fever pneumonia
   Q Fever Hepatitis
   Chronic Q Fever endocarditis

Francisella tularensis
   (some **Vector** transmission)
   Tularemia ascending lymphadenitis

CAT-RELATED

Bartonella henselae
   Cat-Scratch disease
   Bacillary angiomatosis
   Sepsis

Pasteurella multocida
   Acute cellulitis
   Sepsis

Bacillus anthracis

ZOONOTIC

GRAM STAIN:
POS

AEROBIC

EXTRACELLULAR

FEATURES:
- Rods : "**boxcar**-shaped"
- Colonies: gray-white on blood agar.

MOTILITY:
None

CAPSULE & GLYCOCALYX:
- **SPORES:**
Germination requires O_2.
- **Capsule:**
Polypeptide: **D-glutamate.**

EXOTOXINS:
- **Anthrax Toxin** (coded on a plasmid):
   - **Edema Factor (EF):** an adenylate cyclase, causes ↑cAMP.
   - **Lethal Factor (LF):** effects unknown.
   - **Protective Antigen (PA):** mediates binding to epithelium and mediates entry of EF and LF into cells.

CLINICAL:
- **Cutaneous Anthrax:**
   - Symptoms: **round black ulcer** (dime to quarter size) on the skin of extremities or face which develops over a few days and lasts weeks and heals with a permanent scar. Lymphadenopathy may be present but the ulcer is **painless**.
   - **Spores** enter wound, germinate, organism grows and releases **toxins**.
   - Can be **fatal** if untreated.
- **Respiratory Anthrax (Woolsorters Disease):**
   - Rare but rapidly **fatal**.
   - **Host inhales spores** (often found in wool), they germinate in oxygen-rich lungs, grow and release toxins. Systemic consequences.

SOURCE & TRANSMISSION:
- Reservoir for spores: grazing herbivores, contaminated animal skins, wool, goat hair and soil. Textile mills can be a source.
- **Zoonotic transmission** occurs when host contacts an infected animal or when host inhales spores.

VIRULENCE FACTORS:
- **Exotoxins**
- **Spore Formation:** enables survival in extreme and harsh conditions.
- Unique **Polypeptide Capsule:**
   enables *B. anthracis* to escape phagocytosis.

TREATMENT:
- **Penicillin G**
- **Erythromycin** in penicillin allergy.
- The lesion does not get excised.

VACCINE & TOXOID:
- **Vaccine** of killed bacteria toxin components.

HOST DEFENSE & IMMUNITY:
- Antibodies to the peptide capsule.
- Vaccine confers long lasting immunity.

LAB TESTS:
- **Catalase**   **Pos**
- Hemolysis   None
- **Polychrome methylene blue** is used to stain the peptide capsule.

Brucella spp

GRAM STAIN:
NEG

Zoonotic

AEROBIC

INTRACELLULAR

FEATURES:
- **Rods** : coccobacilli.
- **Colonies:** grow very slowly on blood agar (4 weeks).

MOTILITY:
None

CAPSULE & GLYCOCALYX:
Unknown

EXOTOXINS:
None

___

ENDOTOXIN:
- **Lipopolysaccharide** (LPS).

CLINICAL:
- **Brucellosis:**
  - Symptoms: **"enteric fever"** like symptoms similar to typhoid fever. **Systemic infection** with multiple organ manifestation such as **GI tract** disturbances, **hepatosplenomegaly**, endocarditis, and **pulmonary** involvement. **Granuloma** formation is common, especially in the liver and other organs of the RES.
  - Symptoms begin about 1 to 2 months after infection.
  - Symptoms, with treatment, last about 2 weeks to several months.
  - Relapses are possible.
  - Can be **fatal**, especially from "culture negative" **endocarditis**.
- **Undulant Fever:**
  - Symptoms: a **chronic** condition with **"flu-like"** symptoms, **fever** and **severe depression** results when Brucellosis remains untreated (symptoms resemble "chronic fatigue syndrome).

SOURCE & TRANSMISSION:
- **Animals** are reservoirs for *Brucella*, so **zoonotic transmission** occurs via **contact** with farm animals such as cattle, goats, sheep and pigs.
- **Abattoir** workers, **veterinarians** and **farmers** are at risk.
- Transmission may also occur via ingesting **raw milk**.
- Transmission may also occur via accidental **auto-inoculation** by veterinarians attempting to inject vaccine into farm animals.

VIRULENCE FACTORS:
- **Endotoxin**: (O-antigens): provides antigenic variation.
- **Superoxide dismutase** enzyme and other factors enable *Brucella* to survive within phagocytes.

TREATMENT:
- **Doxycycline** (oral) plus **Gentamicin** (IM).
- **TMP-SMZ** plus **Gentamicin** for children or during pregnancy.
- **Prevention:**
  Pasteurization of milk.
  Vaccination of farm animals.

VACCINE & TOXOID:
Vaccine for **animals** only.

HOST DEFENSE & IMMUNITY:
- **IgM** and eventually **IgG** antibodies are used to fight the infection.
- **T-cell** mediated immunity and **cytokines** are important to activate phagocytes and promote intracellular killing.
- Delayed hypersensitivity causes granuloma formation.

LAB TESTS:
●Oxidase	+/-
●**Catalase**	**Pos**
●TSI (H2S)	+/-
●Urease	+/-

Coxiella burnetii

GRAM STAIN:
NEG

Zoonotic

AEROBIC

INTRACELLULAR

FEATURES:
●**Rods** : coccobacilli.
●Colonies: require **cell culture**,
or embryonated eggs,
or test animals.

MOTILITY:
None

CAPSULE & GLYCOCALYX:
●**SPORES:**

EXOTOXINS:
None

ENDOTOXIN:
●**Lipopolysaccharide** (LPS).

CLINICAL:
●**Q Fever: Acute Febrile Illness:**
  ▪Symptoms: **"flu-like"** with **fever**, chills, headache, photophobia and
      chest pain.
  ▪Symptoms begin about 3 weeks after infection.
  ▪Symptoms are self-limited and last about 2 weeks.
  ▪**Note:** very small dose of **less than 10 organisms can cause disease**.
●**Q Fever: Pneumonia:** Atypical Pneumonia.
  ▪Symptoms: interstitial pneumonia with **non-productive cough** and
      inspiratory crackles, fever, chills, headache, and chest pain.
  ▪Symptoms begin about 3 weeks after infection.
  ▪Symptoms last about 1 month
●**Q Fever Hepatitis:**
  ▪Fever and "**doughnut granuloma**" liver biopsy (lipid with fibrin ring).
●**Chronic Q Fever: Acute or Subacute Endocarditis:**
  .▪Symptoms: rare, "culture-negative" endocarditis with nodular valve
      vegetations, hepatosplenomegaly, finger clubbing.
  ▪May be incurable or **fatal**.

SOURCE & TRANSMISSION:
  ●**Animals** are reservoirs for *Coxiella* , so **zoonotic transmission**
  occurs via **contact** with farm animals such as cattle, goats, sheep
  pigs, rabbits, birds, and many other animals.
  ●Transmission may occur via **tick**, **mosquito** and **fly** vectors.
  ●Transmission occurs mostly via **inhalation of contaminated
  aerosols**. *C. burnetii* is found in the urine, feces, milk, and
  placenta of animals, as well as in the nearby soil and dust.
  ●Transmission may occur via ingesting **raw milk.**
  ●**Abattoir** workers, **veterinarians**, and **farmers** are at risk.

VIRULENCE FACTORS:
●**Endotoxin**: (O-antigens): provides antigenic variation.
●**Superoxide dismutase** enzyme and other factors enable *Coxiella* to
      survive within the acidic phagolysosome.
●**Spores:** enable survival in extreme conditions or on fomites or in soil
      for long periods of time.

TREATMENT:
●**Tetracycline** for pneumonia.
●**Doxycycline** plus **TMP-SMZ** (or
plus **Rifampin**) for minimum of 2 yrs,
and **surgical valve replacement** for
endocarditis.
●**Prevention:** pasteurization of milk,
destruction of animal placentas.

VACCINE & TOXOID:

None

HOST DEFENSE & IMMUNITY:
●**IgM** and eventually **IgG** antibodies are
used to fight the infection.
●**T-cell** mediated immunity and **cytokines**
are important to activate phagocytes and
promote intracellular killing.
●Delayed hypersensitivity causes granuloma
formation.

LAB TESTS:
●**Weil-Felix Reaction:**
(Types of Rickettsial-infected
serum can agglutinate strains of
Proteus vulgaris)
  ox-19   Neg
  ox-2   Neg
  ox-K   Neg

Francisella tularensis

GRAM STAIN:
NEG
BIPOLAR STAINING

Zoonotic

AEROBIC

INTRACELLULAR

FEATURES:
- Rods : coccobacilli.
      Bipolar staining.
- Colonies: on cysteine media.
Not usually cultured: **Dangerous.**

MOTILITY:
None

CAPSULE & GLYCOCALYX:
Capsule:
      Lipid

EXOTOXINS:
None

ENDOTOXIN:
- **Lipopolysaccharide** (LPS).

CLINICAL:
- **Tularemia:**
   - Symptoms: **fever**, chills, headache, local or ascending **lymphadenitis** (with tender, swollen lymph nodes), and local skin **ulceration** at the point of entry. Can be **fatal** without proper treatment.
   - Symptoms begin about 5 days after animal contact.
   - Symptoms may last for months.

SOURCE & TRANSMISSION:
- **Animals** are reservoirs for *Francisella*, **zoonotic transmission** occurs via **contact** with many wild animals such as beaver, muskrat, rabbit, squirrel, and sometimes deer.
- Transmission may occur via **tick**, **mosquito** and **fly** vectors.
- Transmission may also occur via contact with contaminated water, or while handling cultures in the laboratory.
- **Hunters** and **trappers** are at risk.

VIRULENCE FACTORS:
- **Endotoxin.**
- **Lipid Capsule:**
   - Provides resistance to phagocytosis
   - Provides resistance to opsonization.

TREATMENT:
- **Streptomycin**

VACCINE & TOXOID:
Live-attenuated:
only for people who are
in contact with animal as
occupation (trappers,
etc.)

HOST DEFENSE & IMMUNITY:
- Antibodies are ineffective.
- **T-cell** mediated immunity and **cytokines** are important to activate phagocytes and promote intracellular killing.
- Previous infection confers long lasting immunity.
- Delayed hypersensitivity causes granuloma formation.

LAB TESTS:
- **Catalase**   Pos

Bartonella henselae formerly *Rochalimaea henselae*

GRAM STAIN:
NEG

Zoonotic

AEROBIC

INTRACELLULAR

FEATURES:
- **Rods**: small, curved.
- Colonies: white and rough mixed with tan, circular; grow very slowly (up to 1 month) on selective media.

MOTILITY:
"twitching"

CAPSULE & GLYCOCALYX:
Unknown

EXOTOXINS:
None

ENDOTOXIN:
- **Lipopolysaccharide (LPS).**

CLINICAL:
- **Cat-Scratch Disease:**
  - Symptoms: local **lymphadenopathy** consisting of tender, swollen lymph nodes (most times just one node); pustules at the scratch site, and sometimes fever.
  - Symptoms begin about two weeks after the scratch.
  - Symptoms may last for months or years.
  - Note: CSD skin test is unsafe and no longer used.
- **Bacillary (epithelioid) Angiomatosis:**
  - Symptoms: proliferative, neovascular **cutaneous** and visceral lesions especially in **immunocompromised** patients. The lesions may be papular and may resemble Kaposi's sarcoma.
- **Bacteremia and Sepsis:**
  - Especially in **immunocompromised** patients.

SOURCE & TRANSMISSION:
- **Cats** are reservoirs for *B. henselae*, usually in their blood.
- **Zoonotic transmission** occurs via being **bit** or **scratched** by the infected **cat** (usually a Kitten).

VIRULENCE FACTORS:
- **Endotoxin**

TREATMENT:
- **Needle aspiration** but no antibiotics for cat-scratch disease.
- **Erythromycin** for bacillary angiomatosis and sepsis.
- **Prevention:** avoid cats in the case of HIV infection.

VACCINE & TOXOID:

None

HOST DEFENSE & IMMUNITY:
- **T-Cell** mediated immunity is important.
- Previous infection confers long lasting immunity.
- Delayed hypersensitivity causes granuloma formation.

LAB TESTS:
- Oxidase   Neg
- Catalase   Neg

Pasteurella multocida

GRAM STAIN:
NEG
BIPOLAR STAINING

Zoonotic

AEROBIC

EXTRACELLULAR

FEATURES:
- **Rods** : coccobacilli.
  Bipolar staining.
- Colonies: gray-yellow, with **musty odor**; on blood agar.

MOTILITY:
None.

CAPSULE & GLYCOCALYX:
Sometimes **Large Capsule**: Polysaccharide.

EXOTOXINS:
None

ENDOTOXIN:
- **Lipopolysaccharide** (LPS).

CLINICAL:
- **Acute Cellulitis:**
  - Symptoms: **rapid** development of local **erythema**, edema and **pain** following animal **bite** or scratch, usually on arm, leg or face.
  - Complications: tendonitis, osteomyelitis, and **abscess formation**.
- **Sepsis:**
  - Caused by spread of local infection to the blood, especially in **immunocompromised** patients.
- Respiratory Diseases:
  - Usually as a complication of underlying chronic respiratory disease.

SOURCE & TRANSMISSION:
- **Animals** are reservoirs for *P. multocida*, usually in their upper respiratory tract and saliva.
- **Zoonotic transmission** occurs via being **bit** or **scratched** by infected animal, especially **cat** or **dog**.
- Transmission may also occur via open wounds which get **licked** by a dog or cat.

VIRULENCE FACTORS:
- **Endotoxin**: (O-antigens): provides antigenic variation.
- **Capsule**: provides protection against phagocytosis.

TREATMENT:
- **Penicillin G** or **ampicillin**.
- **Doxycycline** in penicillin allergy.
- **Prevention:** avoid cats in the case of HIV infection.

VACCINE & TOXOID:

None

HOST DEFENSE & IMMUNITY:
- Strong **acute inflammatory** response with PMNs.
- **IgM** and eventually **IgG** antibodies are used to fight the infection.

LAB TESTS:
Oxidase	+/-
Catalase	**Pos**
Indole	**Pos**
Methyl Red	Neg

Chapter 10

VECTOR-BORNE BACTERIA

VECTOR TRANSMISSION:

Arthropods are vectors.

Animals are reservoirs.

Humans are hosts.

No Subsequent Horizontal or Vertical transmission.

FLEA-BORNE

Yersinia pestis
(Reservoir = rats)
      Bubonic plague
      Septic plague
      Pneumonic plague

Rickettsia typhi
(Reservoir = rats)
      Endemic flea-borne typhus
        (Murine typhus)

LOUSE-BORNE

Bartonella quintana
(Reservoir = humans)
      Trench fever

Rickettsia prowazeckii
(Reservoir = humans)
      Epidemic louse-borne typhus
      Brill-Zinsser disease

Borrelia recurrentis
(Reservoir = humans)
(see Spirochete chapter)
      Relapsing fever

MITE-BORNE

Rickettsia akari
(Reservoir = mice)
      Rickettsial pox

Rickettsia tsutsugamushi
(Reservoir = mice, rodents)
      Mite-borne typhus
        (Scrub typhus)

TICK-BORNE

Ehrlichia chaffeensis
(Reservoir =　　　　)
      Human Ehrlichiosis

Rickettsia rickettsii #1 rickettsial borne.
(Reservoir = dogs, mammals, ticks)
      Rocky mountain spotted fever

Borrelia burgdorferi #1 vector borne.
(Reservoir = deer, mice, ticks)
(see Spirochete chapter)
      Lyme disease

Yersinia pestis

GRAM STAIN:
NEG
BIPOLAR STAINING

Vectors

AEROBIC

INTRACELLULAR

FEATURES:
- **Rods:** coccobacilli.
  Bipolar staining.
- **Colonies:** on blood agar.
Dangerous.

MOTILITY:
None

CAPSULE & GLYCOCALYX:
Capsule:
Protein-polysaccharide.

EXOTOXINS:
Enterotoxin is produced but without significance.

ENDOTOXIN:
- **Lipopolysaccharide** (LPS).

CLINICAL:
- **Bubonic Plague:**
  - Symptoms: **fever**, chills, and **sudden onset** of large, painful **buboes** (femoral, inguinal, axillary or cervical lymphadenitis). **Bacteremia** and **sepsis** may ensue within days to cause high fever, tachycardia, hypotension and complete prostration. **Bubonic purpura** is a cutaneous manifestation of vasculitis which can lead to **gangrene** necrosis (hence **"Black Death"**). Infection is often **fatal within days.**
  - Symptoms arise a few days after the **flea** bite.
  - Symptoms resolve in wks to months with treatment.
- **Septic Plague:**
  - Same symptoms and course as bubonic plague but **no buboes** arise.
- **Pneumonic Plague:** Bronchopneumonia
  - Symptoms: fever, cough with purulent sputum, and hemoptysis.
  - Arises via **hematogenous** spread of *Y. pestis* from buboes, or from inhalation of infected aerosols. Rapid onset and usually **fatal.**.

SOURCE & TRANSMISSION:
- **Animals** are reservoirs for *Y. pestis*, especially **urban rats**, and **sylvatic** (woodland) **rats**, **squirrels**, and **prairie dogs**; **vector transmission** occurs via **flea bite**.
- Transmission may also occur via ingestion of infected animal.
- Rarely, transmission may occur via infected human aerosols or from contact with animals.

VIRULENCE FACTORS:
- **Endotoxin:** (O-antigens): provides antigenic variation.
- **Capsule:** (coded on plasmid)
  - **Envelope antigen F-1:** enhances survival within phagocytes.
- **Enzymes:**
  - **Coagulase:** causes blood to clot during mosquito blood meal.
  - **Fibrinolysin:**
- **Special Requirements:**
  - Calcium.
- Ability to absorb **organic iron** via siderophore-independent means.
- Ability to resist serum complement (coded on plasmid)
- *Y. pestis* has the ability to survive in animal blood and flea gut.

TREATMENT:
- **Streptomycin**
- **IV fluids** and **dopamine** for hypotension and dehydration.
- **Prevention**
Keep patient in isolation.
Rodent control and insecticides.

VACCINE & TOXOID:
Killed bacteria:
used by people who may be at risk: travelers, lab workers, etc.
Boosters every 6 mos.

HOST DEFENSE & IMMUNITY:
- **IgM** and **IgG** antibodies to various bacterial components.
- Strong **acute inflammatory** response with PMNs.
- **T-Cell** mediated immunity is important.
- **Complement** is ineffective.
- **Delayed hypersensitivity** causes granuloma formation.

LAB TESTS:

●Oxidase	Neg
●**Catalase**	**Pos**
●Lactose	Neg
●Indole	+/-
●**Methyl Red**	**Pos**
●Voges-Proskauer	Neg
●Simmon's citrate	+/-
●TSI (H2S)	Neg
●Urease	Neg

Rickettsia typhi

GRAM STAIN:
NEG
(stain poorly)

Vectors

AEROBIC

OBLIGATE INTRACELLULAR

FEATURES:
- **Rods**: coccobacilli.
- Colonies: require **cell culture**, or embryonated eggs, or test animals.

MOTILITY:
None

CAPSULE & GLYCOCALYX:
None

EXOTOXINS:
None

_____

ENDOTOXIN:
- **Lipopolysaccharide** (LPS).

CLINICAL:
- **Endemic Flea-Borne Typhus** (Murine Typhus):
  - *R. typhi* Murine Typhus is a systemic infection which begins when the *R. typhi* enter the bloodstream via a **flea** bite. The rickettsemia progresses to cause **vasculitis** of the small vessels of many organs (especially **liver**) and skin lesions.
  - Symptoms: fever, chills, and **macular rash** mostly on the trunk.
  - Symptoms arise 1-2 weeks after **flea bite**.
  - Symptoms resolve in about 3 weeks, fatalities are rare.
  - **Note:** very small dose of **less than 10 organisms can cause disease**.

SOURCE & TRANSMISSION:
- **Animals** are reservoirs for *R. typhi*, especially **urban** and suburban **rats** and opossums; **vector transmission** occurs during **flea bite**.
(Trans-ovarian transmission from flea to flea offspring occurs.)
- Mostly during **warm** weather in **crowded** conditions.

VIRULENCE FACTORS:
- **Endotoxin**: (O-antigens): provides antigenic variation.
- *R. typhi* has the ability to survive within phagocytes and to **induce** phagocytosis to gain entry into host's **endothelial cells**.
- *R. typhi* has the ability to survive in rat blood and flea feces.
- **Enzyme: Phospholipase A:**
   Causes lysis of phagosomal wall enabling the rickettsiae to escape
   into the host cell's cytoplasm.

TREATMENT:
- **Doxycycline**
- **Chloramphenicol** during pregnancy.
- **Prevention**
Rodent control and insecticides.

VACCINE & TOXOID:
None

HOST DEFENSE & IMMUNITY:
- **IgM** and **IgG** antibodies to various bacterial components.
- **T-Cell** mediated immunity is important.
- Previous infection confers long lasting immunity.
- Cross-immunity against *R. typhi* is provided by previous infection with *R. Prowazekii* (the reverse is not true).

LAB TESTS:
- **Giemsa** or **Gimenez stain**.
- **Weil-Felix Reaction:**
(Types of Rickettsial-infected serum can agglutinate strains of *Proteus vulgaris*)

ox-19	Pos
ox-2	Neg
ox-K	Neg

- Guinea pig testicular swelling.

Bartonella quintana formerly *Rochalimaea quintana*

GRAM STAIN:
NEG

Vectors

AEROBIC

EXTRACELLULAR

FEATURES:
● Rods: small, curved.
●Colonies: tan, circular; grow very slowly (up to 1 month) on selective media.

MOTILITY:
"twitching"

CAPSULE & GLYCOCALYX:
None

EXOTOXINS:
None

ENDOTOXIN:
●**Lipopolysaccharide** (LPS).

CLINICAL:
●**Trench Fever:**
  ▪ *B. quintana*Trench Fever is a systemic infection which results in perivascular inflammation.
  ▪Symptoms: **fever** (may occur in cycles lasting about 5 days), chills, headache, severe **bone pain**, and a **transient rash**.
  ▪Symptoms arise about 2 weeks to 1 month after **louse bite**.
  ▪Symptoms may **relapse** many times over months or years, but the infection is most often self-limited after 2 months.
  ▪**Note:** very small dose of **less than 10 organisms can cause disease**.

SOURCE & TRANSMISSION:
●**Humans** are the only reservoirs for *B. quintana*; **vector transmission** occurs during **louse bite**.
●Mostly during **cold** weather (lice infest clothing) in **crowded** conditions, or during **wartime**.
●Transmission also occurs via inhalation of lice-feces-aerosol dust from clothing of infected patients.
●**Epidemics** may occur.

VIRULENCE FACTORS:
●**Endotoxin**
● *B. quintana* has the ability to survive in human blood and louse feces.

TREATMENT:
●**Doxycycline**
●**Erythromycin** during pregnancy.
●**Prevention**
Insecticides.

VACCINE & TOXOID:

None

HOST DEFENSE & IMMUNITY:
●**IgM** and **IgG** antibodies to various bacterial components.

LAB TESTS:
●Oxidase   Neg
●Catalase   Neg

Rickettsia prowazeckii

GRAM STAIN:
NEG
(stain poorly)

Vectors

AEROBIC

OBLIGATE INTRACELLULAR

FEATURES:
● **Rods**: coccobacilli.
●Colonies: require **cell culture**,
or embryonated eggs,
or test animals.

MOTILITY:
None

CAPSULE & GLYCOCALYX:
None

EXOTOXINS:
None

ENDOTOXIN:
●**Lipopolysaccharide** (LPS).

CLINICAL:
●**Epidemic Louse-Borne Typhus:**
■ *R. prowazeckii* Epidemic Typhus is a systemic infection which begins
when the *R. prowazeckii* enter the bloodstream via a **louse** bite.
The rickettsemia progresses to cause **vasculitis** of the small
vessels of many organs (especially **liver**), skin lesions, and
clotting abnormalities.
■Symptoms: **high fever**, chills, and **macular rash** mostly on the trunk.
The rash eventually becomes papular or **petechial**, coalesces
and spreads **centrifugally** to involve the whole body **except**
the face, palms, and soles.
■Symptoms arise 1 week after **louse bite**.
■Symptoms resolve in about 2 weeks, but complete recovery may take
months, can be **fatal**.
■**Note:** very small dose of **less than 10 organisms can cause disease**.
●**Brill-Zinsser Disease:**
■Recrudescent epidemic typhus.
■Occurs months to years after recovery from initial infection.

SOURCE & TRANSMISSION:
●**Humans** and **flying squirrels** are reservoirs for *R. Prowazekii*;
vector transmission occurs during **louse bite**.
●Mostly during **cold** weather (lice infest clothing) in **crowded**
conditions, or during wartime.
●Transmission also occurs via inhalation of lice-feces-aerosol
dust from clothing of infected patients.
●**Epidemics** may occur.

VIRULENCE FACTORS:
●**Endotoxin**: (O-antigens): provides antigenic variation.
●*R. Prowazekii* has the ability to survive within phagocytes and to **induce**
phagocytosis to gain entry into host's **endothelial cells**.
●*R. Prowazekii* has the ability to survive in human blood and louse feces.
●**Enzyme: Phospholipase A:**
Causes lysis of phagosomal wall enabling the rickettsiae to escape
into the host cell's cytoplasm.

TREATMENT:
●**Doxycycline**
●**Chloramphenicol** during pregnancy.
●**Prevention**
Insecticides.

VACCINE & TOXOID:
Killed bacteria:
for people who may be at
risk: travelers, lab workers,
and the patients' care-takers.

HOST DEFENSE & IMMUNITY:
●**IgM** and **IgG** antibodies to various
bacterial components.
●**T-Cell** mediated immunity is important.
●**Cross-immunity** against *R. typhi* is
provided by previous infection with
R. Prowazekii (the reverse is not true).

LAB TESTS:
●**Giemsa** or **Gimenez stain**.
●**Weil-Felix Reaction:**
(Types of Rickettsial-infected
serum can agglutinate strains of
Proteus vulgaris)

ox-19	**Pos**
ox-2	Neg
ox-K	Neg

Rickettsia akari

GRAM STAIN:
NEG
(stain poorly)

Vectors

AEROBIC

OBLIGATE INTRACELLULAR

FEATURES:
● **Rods:** coccobacilli.
●Colonies: require **cell culture**,
or embryonated eggs,
or test animals.

MOTILITY:

None

CAPSULE & GLYCOCALYX:

None

EXOTOXINS:
None

ENDOTOXIN:
●**Lipopolysaccharide** (LPS).

CLINICAL:
●**Rickettsial Pox:**
- *R. akari* Rickettsial Pox is a systemic infection which begins when the *R. akari* enter the bloodstream via a mouse-**mite bite**. The rickettsemia progresses to cause **vasculitis** of small vessels and skin lesions.
- Symptoms: a **papule** develops at the bite-site then ulcerates to form an **eschar** (a dark scab). Rapid onset of **fever**, chills, headache, **photophobia**, and myalgia sometimes with mild, non-tender local lymphadenopathy; then a general **papulo-vesicular** rash appears.
- Symptoms arise 1 week after **mite bite**; papule and eschar occur first; after another 2 weeks, the other symptoms arise.
- Symptoms resolve in about 3 weeks after pox-like lesions appear; disease is **self-limited.**
- **Note:** very small dose of **less than 10 organisms can cause disease.**

SOURCE & TRANSMISSION:
●**Mice** are reservoirs for *R. akari*, **vector transmission** occurs during **mite bite**.
(Trans-ovarian transmission from mite to mite offspring occurs.)
●During **warm** weather.

VIRULENCE FACTORS:
●**Endotoxin:** (O-antigens): provides antigenic variation.
● *R. akari* has the ability to survive within phagocytes and to **induce** phagocytosis to gain entry into host's **endothelial cells**.
● *R. akari* has the ability to survive in mouse blood and in mites.
●**Enzyme: Phospholipase A:**
Causes lysis of phagosomal wall enabling the rickettsiae to escape into the host cell's cytoplasm.

TREATMENT:
●**Doxycycline** to speed recovery.
●**Chloramphenicol** during pregnancy.
●**Prevention**
Rodent control and insecticides.

VACCINE & TOXOID:

None

HOST DEFENSE & IMMUNITY:
●**IgM** and **IgG** antibodies to various bacterial components.
●**T-Cell** mediated immunity is important.

LAB TESTS:
●**Giemsa** or **Gimenez stain**.
●**Weil-Felix Reaction:**
(Types of Rickettsial-infected serum can agglutinate strains of *Proteus vulgaris*)
ox-19   Neg
ox-2   Neg
ox-K   Neg

Rickettsia tsutsugamushi

GRAM STAIN:
NEG
(stain poorly)

Vectors

AEROBIC

OBLIGATE INTRACELLULAR

FEATURES:
- **Rods**: coccobacilli.
- Colonies: require **cell culture**, or embryonated eggs, or test animals.

MOTILITY:
None

CAPSULE & GLYCOCALYX:
None

EXOTOXINS:
None

___

ENDOTOXIN:

NOTE: No endotoxin.

CLINICAL:
- **Scrub Typhus (Mite-Borne Typhus):**
  - *R. tsutsugamushi* Scrub Typhus is a systemic infection which begins when the *R. tsutsugamushi* enter the bloodstream via a rodent **mite larva bite** (chigger). The rickettsemia progresses to cause **vasculitis** of small vessels and skin lesions.
  - Rare in the United States, more common in **Asia.**
  - Symptoms: a **papule** develops at the bite-site then ulcerates to form an **eschar** (a dark scab). Rapid onset of **high fever**, chills, headache, and myalgia with **tender local lymphadenopathy**; then a **maculo-papular** rash appears on the **trunk** and spreads **centrifugally** to the extremities.
  - Symptoms arise 1-2 weeks after **mite-chigger bite**; papule and eschar occur first; after another 5 days, the other symptoms arise.
  - Symptoms resolve in about 2 weeks after skin lesions appear; disease is often **self-limited**, but it can be **fatal.**
  - **Note:** very small dose of **less than 10 organisms can cause disease.**

SOURCE & TRANSMISSION:
- **Rodents** are reservoirs for *R. tsutsugamushi*; **vector transmission** occurs during **mite larva bite** (chiggers) (Trans-ovarian transmission from mite to mite offspring occurs.)
- During **warm** weather.

VIRULENCE FACTORS:
- Many serotypes.
- *R. tsutsugamushi* has the ability to survive within phagocytes and to **induce** phagocytosis to gain entry into host's **endothelial cells.**
- *R. tsutsugamushi* has the ability to survive in mouse blood and in mites.
- **Enzyme: Phospholipase A:**
  Causes lysis of phagosomal wall enabling the rickettsiae to escape into the host cell's cytoplasm.

TREATMENT:
- **Doxycycline** to speed recovery.
- **Chloramphenicol** during pregnancy.
- **Prevention**
Rodent control and insecticides.

VACCINE & TOXOID:

None

HOST DEFENSE & IMMUNITY:
- **IgM** and **IgG** antibodies to various bacterial components.
- **T-Cell** mediated immunity is important.

LAB TESTS:
- **Giemsa** or **Gimenez stain.**
- **Weil-Felix Reaction:**
(Types of Rickettsial-infected serum can agglutinate strains of *Proteus vulgaris*)

ox-19	Neg
ox-2	Neg
ox-K	**Pos** (some Neg)

Ehrlichia chaffeensis

GRAM STAIN:
NEG
(stain poorly)

Vectors

AEROBIC

OBLIGATE INTRACELLULAR

FEATURES:
● **Rods**: coccobacilli.
●Colonies: require **cell culture**,
not usually done.

MOTILITY:

None

CAPSULE & GLYCOCALYX:

None

EXOTOXINS:
None

ENDOTOXIN:

NOTE: No endotoxin.

CLINICAL:
●**Human Ehrlichiosis:**
- *E. chaffeensis* Ehrlichiosis is a systemic infection which begins when the *E. chaffeensis* enter the bloodstream and lymphatics via a **tick** bite. The Ehrlichemia progresses to cause multi-organ dysfunction, but **no vasculitis**.
- Symptoms: slow onset of **fever**, headache, chills, myalgia, nausea and anorexia; then a **maculo-papular** rash may or may not appear. Disease may progress to **leukopenia**, **pulmonary failure**, **renal failure**, **encephalitis**; and it can be **fatal**.
- Poor prognosis when infection occurs in the elderly.
- Symptoms arise 1 week after **tick bite**.
- Symptoms resolve in several weeks, or more rapidly with treatment.

SOURCE & TRANSMISSION:
●Reservoir for *E. chaffeensis* is unknown; **vector transmission** occurs during **tick bite** .
●During **warm** weather.

VIRULENCE FACTORS:
● *E. chaffeensis* has the ability to survive within Macros.
● *E. chaffeensis* has the ability to survive in ticks.

TREATMENT:
●**Doxycycline**
●**Prevention**
Prompt removal of ticks.

VACCINE & TOXOID:

None

HOST DEFENSE & IMMUNITY:
●**IgM** and **IgG antibodies** to various bacterial components and **complement** are effective to help clear the bacteria.
● *E. chaffeensis* can survive in **Macros** but not in **PMNs**.

LAB TESTS:
●**Peripheral blood smear** shows cytoplasmic inclusion vacuole (**"morulae"** filled with bacteria) inside granulocytes.
●**Serology** shows increased titer for *E. chaffeensis* antibody.

Rickettsia rickettsii

GRAM STAIN:
NEG
(stain poorly)

Vectors

AEROBIC

OBLIGATE INTRACELLULAR

FEATURES:
● **Rods**: coccobacilli.
●Colonies: require **cell culture**,
or embryonated eggs,
or test animals.

MOTILITY:
None

CAPSULE & GLYCOCALYX:
None

EXOTOXINS:
None

ENDOTOXIN:
●Lipopolysaccharide (LPS).

CLINICAL:
●**Rocky Mountain Spotted Fever:**
▪ *R. rickettsii* Rocky Mountain Spotted Fever is a systemic infection
which begins when the *R. rickettsii* enter the bloodstream via
a **tick** bite. The rickettsemia progresses to cause **vasculitis** of
small vessels of many organs (especially **lungs**), skin lesions,
and fulminant disease.
▪**Most common Rickettsial disease in the United States**.
▪Symptoms: often there is no mark noticed at the bite site. Rapid onset
of **high fever**, headache, nausea, **vomiting**, and myalgia; then
a **maculo-papular** rash appears on the wrists, **palms** and **soles**.
The rash may become **petechial** then necrotic and gangrenous.
Disease may progress to **pulmonary failure**, **renal failure**,
encephalitis and coma; and it can be **rapidly fatal**.
▪Worst prognosis in the elderly, in males, and in G6PD deficiency.
▪Symptoms arise 1 week after **tick bite**; fever and nausea occur first;
after another 5 days, the rash begins.
▪Symptoms resolve in about 3 weeks with **early aggressive treatment**.
▪**Note:** very small dose of **less than 10 organisms can cause disease**.

SOURCE & TRANSMISSION:
●**Animals** and **ticks** are reservoirs for *R. rickettsii*, **vector
transmission** occurs during **tick bite** (tick must remain attached
for 6-8 hours or longer).
(Trans-ovarian transmission from tick to tick offspring occurs.)
●During **warm** weather.

VIRULENCE FACTORS:
●**Endotoxin**: (O-antigens): provides antigenic variation.
● *R. rickettsii* has the ability to survive within phagocytes and to **induce**
phagocytosis to gain entry into host's **endothelial cells**.
● *R. rickettsii* has the ability to survive in animal blood and in ticks.
●**Enzyme: Phospholipase A:**
Causes lysis of phagosomal wall enabling the rickettsiae to escape
into the host cell's cytoplasm.

TREATMENT:
●**Doxycycline** must be administered
very early in the course of disease.
●Admission to **ICU** may be necessary.
●**Chloramphenicol** during pregnancy.
●**Prevention**
Rodent control, insecticides, and
prompt removal of ticks.

VACCINE & TOXOID:
None

HOST DEFENSE & IMMUNITY:
●**IgM** and **IgG** antibodies to various
bacterial components.
●**T-Cell** mediated immunity is important.
●Previous infection confers long lasting
immunity.

LAB TESTS:
●**Giemsa** or **Gimenez** stain.
●**Weil-Felix Reaction:**
(Types of Rickettsial-infected
serum can agglutinate strains of
Proteus vulgaris)
ox-19　**Pos**
ox-2　**Pos**
ox-K　Neg

Chapter 11

GRAM POSITIVE ACID-FAST AND MODIFIED ACID-FAST BACTERIA

TUBERCULOUS MYCOBACTERIUM	NONTUBERCULOUS MYCOBACTERIUM	MODIFIED ACID-FAST	LEPROSY
Mycobacterium tuberculosis 　　Primary tuberculosis 　　Secondary tuberculosis 　　Miliary tuberculosis 　　Extra-pulmonary tuberculosis 　　　　Pott's disease (skeletal) 　　　　Chronic meningitis 　　　　Scrofuloderma (skin) 　　Tuberculosis and AIDS *Mycobacterium bovis* (Zoonotic) 　　Pulmonary tuberculosis 　　Extra-pulmonary tuberculosis 　　　　GI tract 　　　　Scrofuloderma (skin)	*Mycobacterium avium-intracellulare complex* 　　MAI pulmonary disease in AIDS **Non-Tuberculous** *Mycobacterium* 　　**Group I:** 　　　　*M. kansasii* 　　　　*M. marinum* 　　**Group II:** 　　　　*M. scrofulaceum* 　　**Group III:** 　　　　MAI 　　**Group IV:** 　　　　*M. smegmatis* 　　　　*M. abscessus* 　　　　*M. chelonei* 　　　　*M. fortuitum*	*Nocardia asteroides* 　　Nocardosis 　　　　Pulmonary abscess 　　　　Sepsis 　　　　Brain abscess 　　Mycetoma	*Mycobacterium leprae* 　　Tuberculoid leprosy 　　Lepromatous leprosy 　　Borderline leprosy

Mycobacterium tuberculosis

GRAM STAIN:
POS
(stains poorly)

ZIEHL-NEELSEN OR KINYOUN STAIN:
ACID FAST
("Alcohol Acid-Fast")

OBLIGATE AEROBE

INTRACELLULAR

FEATURES:
- **Rods** : grow in **cords**.
- Colonies: very slow growth on special media.

MOTILITY:
None

CAPSULE & GLYCOCALYX:
Complex **lipid** and **polypeptide** coat.

EXOTOXINS:
None

ENDOTOXIN:
None

CLINICAL:
- **PPD Positive:**
    - Indicates exposure to *M. tuberculosis* and intact T-cell response.
    - May be permanently inactive and asymptomatic.
- **Primary Tuberculosis:**
    - *M. tuberculosis* lodges initially in **lower lobe** of lung.
    - **Tubercle formation: granuloma** of *M. tuberculosis* inside Macros; surrounded by Langhans cells, epithelioid cells, and Lymphos. Central area may undergo **caseating necrosis** or **calcification**. *M. tuberculosis* may survive for many years like this.
    - **Ghon complex** = primary tubercle plus associated swollen lymph node. Shows well on **chest x-ray**.
- **Secondary Tuberculosis:**
    - *M. tuberculosis* **reactivates** in **upper lobe** due to higher oxygenation.
    - This active form of disease usually results from **impaired immunity**.
    - **Sputum** smear becomes acid-fast POS, **cavitating** lesions may occur.
    - Infection may spread by **local extension** to nearby tissues.
    - Disease becomes **contagious**.
- **Miliary Tuberculosis:**
    - Widespread **hematological dissemination** of *M. tuberculosis* results in "shot-gun pellet" type lesion in lungs, CNS, GI tract, kidney, or almost any other organ, including the bones.
- **Extra-pulmonary TB:**
    Pott's Disease (skeletal); Chronic **meningitis**; scrofuloderma (skin); etc.
- **Tuberculosis in AIDS:**
    - Fulminant course and more extra-pulmonary symptoms.
    - PPD may become NEG due to weak cellular immunity.
- **TB causes more world-wide fatalities than any other infectious disease.**

SOURCE & TRANSMISSION:
- **Humans** are the only reservoirs, and horizontal transmission occurs via **respiratory droplets** from actively infected person.
- Rare horizontal transmission may occur via skin contact (scrofuloderma), especially to pathologists during autopsies

VIRULENCE FACTORS:
- **Cord Factor** (trehalose dimycolate): gathers *M. tuberculosis* in chains.
- **Abundant Peptide Antigens** of outer coat:
    - **Stimulate actively self-destructive host immunity.**
    - NOTE: There are no enzymes or toxins to cause destruction.
- **Isoniazid Resistance:** (Note: Isoniazid requires catalase for its activation)
    - Random **mutation** occurs to cause **loss of catalase activity**.
- *M. tuberculosis* produces substances to allow **survival within Macros**.
- *M. tuberculosis* survives **acidic**, **alkaline**, or **drying** conditions.
- **Lipid-rich** cell wall (mycolic acid, wax D, etc.) **resists disinfectants**.

TREATMENT:
- **Isoniazid (INH)** for PPD POS; for HIV POS prophylaxis; for contacts of active TB.
- **Multi-Drug Therapy:**
    1. **Isoniazid plus Vitamin B6**
    2. **Rifampin** (or Ketoconazole if on birth control)
    3. **Pyrazinamide**
    4. Streptomycin or Ethambutol (not in pregnancy) (not in children)
- **Warning:** use of immunosupressive drugs (e.g. steroids) can re-activate TB.
- **Isolation** may be necessary.

VACCINE & TOXOID:
BCG Vaccine: Live attenuated bacteria. Does not stop infection. **Not available in USA.**

HOST DEFENSE & IMMUNITY:
- **T-cell** mediated **delayed hypersensitivity**.
- Antibodies are ineffective.
- **Cytokines** are important to activate both Lymphos and Macros; this enhances the intracellular killing of *M. tuberculosis*.
- **Macrophages** fuse to form **Langhans Giant Cells**.
- **Granulomas** form with **epithelioid** cells surrounding central **necrosis**.

LAB TESTS:
- Acid-fast stain of sputum smear.
- Culture of sputum.
- Chest X-Ray.
- **PPD skin test (Mantaux):** Inject TB antigen sub-dermally and check at **48-72 hrs**:
    - **Induration >10 mm = POS.**
    - Redness or induration **< 5mm** = NEG.
    - Induration **5mm-10 mm** indicates immunocompromised state
- **Catalase   POS**
- **Generate Niacin.**
- No pigment production.
- **Nitrate reduction.**

Mycobacterium bovis

GRAM STAIN:
POS
(stains poorly)

ZIEHL-NEELSEN OR KINYOUN STAIN:
ACID FAST
("**Alcohol** Acid-Fast")

ZOONOTIC

OBLIGATE AEROBE

INTRACELLULAR

FEATURES:
- **Rods** : grow in **cords**.
- Colonies: very slow growth on special media.

MOTILITY:
None

CAPSULE & GLYCOCALYX:
Complex **lipid** and **polypeptide** coat.

EXOTOXINS:
None

ENDOTOXIN:
None

CLINICAL:
- *M. bovis* **Tuberculosis:**
  - Causes **GI tract** infection, **pulmonary** infection, and scrofuloderma.
  - Very **rare** in the USA.

SOURCE & TRANSMISSION:
- **Mammals** are the only reservoirs, **zoonotic transmission** occurs via ingestion of **raw milk** from infected animal.
- Horizontal transmission occurs via **respiratory droplets**.
- Rare horizontal transmission may occur via skin contact (scrofuloderma), especially to pathologists during autopsies
- Infection occur in underdeveloped nations and in San Diego.

VIRULENCE FACTORS:
- **Abundant Peptide Antigens** of outer coat:
  - **Stimulate actively self-destructive host immunity.**
  - NOTE: There are no enzymes or toxins to cause destruction.
- **Isoniazid Resistance:** (Note: Isoniazid requires catalase for its activation)
  - Random **mutation** occurs to cause **loss of catalase activity**.
- *M. bovis* produces substances to allow **survival within Macros**.
- *M. bovis* survives **acidic**, **alkaline**, or **drying** conditions.
- **Lipid-rich** cell wall (mycolic acid, wax D, etc.) **resists disinfectants**.

TREATMENT:
- **Isoniazid (INH)** for PPD POS;
  for HIV POS prophylaxis;
  for contacts of active TB.
- **Multi-Drug Therapy:**
  1. **Isoniazid plus Vitamin B6**
  2. **Rifampin** (or Ketoconazole if on birth control)
  3. **Pyrazinamide**
  4. Streptomycin or Ethambutol
     (not in pregnancy)
     (not in children)
- **Warning:** use of immunosupressive drugs (e.g. steroids) can re-activate TB.
- **Isolation** may be necessary.

VACCINE & TOXOID:
BCG Vaccine:
Live attenuated bacteria.
Does not stop infection.
Used only for farm animals in USA.

HOST DEFENSE & IMMUNITY:
- **T-cell** mediated **delayed hypersensitivity**.
- Antibodies are ineffective.
- **Cytokines** are important to activate both Lymphos and Macros; this enhances the intracellular killing of *M. bovis* .
- Macrophages fuse to form **Langhans Giant Cells**.
- **Granulomas** form with **epithelioid** cells surrounding central **necrosis**.

LAB TESTS:
- Acid-fast stain of sputum smear.
- Culture of sputum.
- Chest X-Ray.
- **PPD skin test:**   **POS**
- Catalase   NEG
- Does not generate Niacin.
- No pigment production.
- No Nitrate reduction.

Mycobacterium avium-intracellulare complex

GRAM STAIN:
POS
(stains poorly)

ZIEHL-NEELSEN OR KINYOUN STAIN:
ACID FAST
("**Alcohol** Acid-Fast")

OBLIGATE AEROBE

INTRACELLULAR

FEATURES:
- **Rods** :
- Colonies: very slow growth on special media.

MOTILITY:
None

CAPSULE & GLYCOCALYX:
Complex **lipid** and **polypeptide** coat.

EXOTOXINS:
None
_____

ENDOTOXIN:
None

CLINICAL:
- MAI **Pulmonary infection:**
  - This a **very common infection** among **AIDS** patients.
  - Causes disease mostly in AIDS patients with **CD4+ count < 100.**
  - MAI causes **pulmonary disease** similar to TB.
    Can lead to cavitation or infiltration.
  - MAI infection quickly **disseminates** to cause lesions in every organ.
    The GI tract is very often involved.
    The lesions are **granulomas** with Macros filled with organisms.
  - MAI infection is usually **fatal** within months.
  - Infection is very difficult to distinguish from TB; **cultures** must be
    made from sputum or blood; then **DNA probes** must be used.

SOURCE & TRANSMISSION:
- MAI organisms are **ubiquitous** in nature and cause disease by **opportunistic infections** in birds and **immunocompromised** humans, especially **AIDS** patients with low CD4 + T cell count.

VIRULENCE FACTORS:
- MAI are low-virulent organisms that cause opportunistic infections.
- **Isoniazid Resistance:** (Note: Isoniazid requires catalase for its activation)
  - Resistant strains of MAI do **not produce catalase.**
- **Multiple Drug Resistance.**
- MAI organisms produce substances to allow **survival within Macros.**
- MAI organisms survive **acidic**, **alkaline**, or **drying** conditions.

TREATMENT:
- **Multi-Drug Therapy:**
  1. **Rifampin**
  2. **Ethambutol**
  3. **Streptomycin**
- Add **Clarithromycin** instead of Streptomycin for disseminated disease.
- **Rifabutin** prophylaxis in **AIDS** at CD4 count < 100.

VACCINE & TOXOID:

None

HOST DEFENSE & IMMUNITY:
- **T-cell** mediated **delayed hypersensitivity.**
- Antibodies are ineffective.
- **Cytokines** are important to activate both Lymphos and Macros; this enhances the intracellular killing of MAI.
- Macrophages fuse to form **Langhans Giant Cells.**
- **Granulomas** form with **epithelioid** cells surrounding central **necrosis.**

LAB TESTS:
- Acid-fast stain of sputum smear.
- Culture of sputum.
- Chest X-Ray.
- Sometimes PPD test POS.
- Catalase   NEG
- Does not generate Niacin.
- No pigment production.
- No Nitrate reduction.

Nontuberculous Mycobacterium spp (NTM)

GRAM STAIN:
POS
(stains poorly)

ZIEHL-NEELSEN OR KINYOUN STAIN:
ACID FAST
("**Alcohol** Acid-Fast")

OBLIGATE AEROBE

INTRACELLULAR

FEATURES:
● Rods:
●Colonies: very slow growth on special media; except Group IV, which grows rapidly.

MOTILITY:
None

CAPSULE & GLYCOCALYX:
Complex **lipid** and **polypeptide** coat.

EXOTOXINS:
None

ENDOTOXIN:
None

CLINICAL:
●**Group I: Photochromogens:** produce yellow pigment upon exposure to light.
  ▪*M. kansasii*: causes **pulmonary** infection similar to TB.
  ▪*M. marinum*: causes "**swimming pool granuloma**" at abrasion site.
●**Group II: Scotochromogens:** produce yellow pigment in the dark.
  ▪*M. scrofulaceum*: causes **Scrofula** (cervical lymphadenitis).
●**Group III: Non-chromogens:** produce no pigments.
  ▪MAI = *M. avium-intracellulare* **complex**: see previous page.
●**Group IV: Non-chromogen, rapid growers**.
  ▪*M. smegmatis*: collects under penis foreskin as **smegma**.
  ▪*M. abscessus, M. chelonei, M. fortuitum*: cause **wound infections**.

SOURCE & TRANSMISSION:
●These **atypical** *Mycobacteria* are **ubiquitous** in nature (soil and water), and cause **opportunistic** infections primarily in **immunocompromised** patients.

VIRULENCE FACTORS:
●These are low-virulent organisms that cause opportunistic infections.
●**Isoniazid Resistance:** (Note: Isoniazid requires catalase for its activation)
  ▪**Resistant strains do not produce catalase**.
●**Multiple Drug Resistance**.
●These produce substances to allow **survival within Macros**.
●These survive **acidic**, **alkaline**, or **drying** conditions.

TREATMENT:
●**Group I:**
M. kansasii: same treatment as TB.
M. marinum: Rifampin + Ethambutol
●**Group II:**
M. scrofulaceum: same treatment as TB
●**Group III:**
see MAI on previous page.
●**Group IV:**
M. smegmatis: Amikacin
M. abscessus, M. chelonei, and *M. fortuitum*: Amikacin + Cefoxitin

VACCINE & TOXOID:
None

HOST DEFENSE & IMMUNITY:
●**T-cell** mediated **delayed hypersensitivity**.
●Antibodies are ineffective.
●**Cytokines** are important to activate both Lymphos and Macros; this enhances the intracellular killing.

LAB TESTS:
●Acid-fast stain of sputum smear.
●Culture of sputum.
●Chest X-Ray.
●Sometimes PPD test POS.
●Catalase   +/-
●Do not generate Niacin.
●**Pigment production**: as noted
●Nitrate reduction   +/-
●Sometimes PPD test POS.

Nocardia asteroides

GRAM STAIN:
POS

MODIFIED ZIEHL-NEELSEN STAIN:
MODIFIED ACID FAST
("Non-Alcohol Acid-Fast")

AEROBIC

EXTRACELLULAR

FEATURES:
● Coccoid Rod: grows in **branched**
filamentous chains
● Colonies: pigmented or not;

MOTILITY:
None

CAPSULE & GLYCOCALYX:
Unknown

EXOTOXINS:
None

ENDOTOXIN:
None

CLINICAL:
● Nocardosis:
▪ Pulmonary Abscesses:
May cause cavitating lesions; may resemble TB.
▪ Septic Nocardosis:
Spreads from pulmonary lesions; may spread to any organ.
▪ Brain Abscesses:
Result from disseminated infection.
▪ Not contagious.
▪ Disease can be **fatal**; or may **relapse** after effective treatment.
● Mycetoma: ("aerobic actinomyces")
▪ Caused by *N. asteroides* in combination with others of *Nocardia spp.*
▪ This is a **chronic granulomatous** infection of **sub-cutaneous** tissues.
▪ **Sinus-tract formation** occurs with draining **pus** open on skin.
▪ **Foot** is the usual site of infection, due to **trauma**.

SOURCE & TRANSMISSION:
● *N. asteroides* organisms are **ubiquitous** in **soil** and cause
opportunistic infections in **immunocompromised** humans,
especially **AIDS** patients with low CD4 + T cell count, and
especially any patient on **corticosteroid** medication.
● The **route** of infection is **respiratory** or **skin trauma**.

VIRULENCE FACTORS:
● Enzymes:
▪ **Catalase** and **Superoxide Dismutase** enable *N. asteroides* to
resist the PMN intracellular oxidative burst.
● **Filament** formation enables *N. asteroides* to resist phagocytosis.

TREATMENT:
● Sulfonamide
● TMP-SMZ prophylaxis
in organ transplant patients taking
immunosupressive medication.
● Amikacin plus Impenem
in sulfa allergy.
● Debridement of mycetoma.

VACCINE & TOXOID:
None

HOST DEFENSE & IMMUNITY:
● **Acute pyogenic inflammation** with **PMN**
phagocytosis is the primary host reaction.
● **Antibodies** are necessary to defend against
the filamentous form of *N. asteroides*.
● **Cytokines** are important to activate both
phagocytes and T-cells.
● Activated **CD8+ T-cells** are capable of
killing *N. asteroides* directly.

LAB TESTS:
● **Modified Ziehl-Neelsen stain**
of **sputum** smear or **pus** smear.
● **Gram stain** of biopsy.
● Culture.
● **Catalase**   POS
● Pigment production: +/-

Mycobacterium leprae

GRAM STAIN:
POS
(stains poorly)

FITE STAIN:
ACID FAST

OBLIGATE AEROBE

INTRACELLULAR

FEATURES:
- **Rods** : in "**globi**" bundles: encapsulated globs of rods in tissue.
- Colonies:
NEVER on artificial media.
Grows only on **foot pad** of Mice.

MOTILITY:

None

CAPSULE & GLYCOCALYX:
Complex **lipid** and **polypeptide** coat.

EXOTOXINS:
None

ENDOTOXIN:
None

CLINICAL:
- **Tuberculoid Leprosy:** (associated with HLA-DR3 genotype)
  - Symptoms:
    Well-defined asymmetrical **cutaneous macular rash** with **erythematous borders** and **pigment loss in center**; associated with areas of **sensory loss** (fine touch, pain, temperature).
  - **Disfigurement** due to trauma, secondary to **sensory loss**.
  - Symptoms, except sensory loss, resolve with treatment but may relapse.
  - Incubation after respiratory transmission is 3-6 years.
  - Biopsy of lesion shows **few** *M. leprae* organisms.
  - **Lepromin** skin test **POS**.
- **Lepromatous Leprosy:** (associated with HLA-MTI genotype)
  - Symptoms:
    Symmetrical cutaneous nodular lesions associated with areas of **sensory loss** (fine touch, pain, temperature) and concurrent **upper respiratory congestion**. Widespread dissemination is due to *M. leprae* specific **immune anergy**.
  - **Disfigurement** due to trauma, secondary to **sensory loss**, especially along ulnar nerve, hands, feet, nose, ears, eyes, and testes.
  - Symptoms, except sensory loss and severe disfigurement, resolve with treatment but may relapse.
  - Incubation after respiratory transmission is 3-10 years.
  - Biopsy of lesion shows **many** *M. leprae* organisms.
  - **Lepromin** skin test **NEG**.
- **Borderline Leprosy:**
  - Most patients have mixture of Tuberculoid and Lepromatous forms.

SOURCE & TRANSMISSION:
- **Humans** and **nine-banded armadillos** are the only reservoirs for *M. leprae*; horizontal transmission occurs via **respiratory droplets** due to **close personal contact**.
- Other routes of transmission suspected: direct contact via skin trauma, zoonotic from armadillos, and vector-borne routes.

VIRULENCE FACTORS:
- **PGL-1 (phenolic glycolipid 1) Capsule:**
  - Scavenges free radicals.
  - Enables *M. leprae* to survive phagocytosis.
- **Lipoarabinomannan glycoprotein** plus PGL-1:
  - Cause immunologic anergy in host.
- Preference for **lower temperature**:
  - Limits infection to **skin** and **naso-pharynx**.
- **Intracellular Survival** within:
  - **Skin histiocytes**.
  - **Schwann cells**.

TREATMENT:
- **Emotional** support.
- **Multi-Drug Therapy:**
  1. **Dapsone**
  2. **Rifampin**
  3. **Clofazimine** is added for Lepromatous form
- Treatment lasts for **many years**.

VACCINE & TOXOID:
BCG Vaccine:
Live attenuated bacteria.
Does not stop infection.
Not available in USA.
Questionable efficacy.

HOST DEFENSE & IMMUNITY:
- **Tuberculoid form:**
  - Weak antibody response.
  - **Cytokines** are important.
  - T-cell mediated **delayed hypersensitivity**.
  - Macros form **Langhans Giant Cells**.
  - **Granulomas** form with **epithelioid** cells.
- **Lepromatous form:**
  - Strong antibody response
  - Weak production of cytokines.
  - *M. leprae* specific **T-cell** immune **anergy**.
  - *M. leprae* specific **Macrophage anergy**.

LAB TESTS:
- **Lepromin Skin test:**
  POS in Tuberculoid form:
      (induration at 3-4 weeks)
  NEG in Lepromatous form.
- Serology test for PGL-1
- **FITE** Acid-fast stain of biopsy.
- Loss of acid-fastness by Pyridine extraction.
- Catalase   NEG
- **Dopa-oxidase POS**
- Does not generate Niacin.
- No pigment production.
- No Nitrate reduction.

Chapter 12

SPIROCHETES

TREPONEMA

Treponema pallidum
        Primary syphilis
        Secondary syphilis
        Latent syphilis
        Secondary syphilis relapse
        Tertiary syphilis
        Congenital syphilis

Treponema pallidum-endemicum
        Bejel
        (oral lesions in children)

Treponema carateum
        Pinta
        (hypopigmenting skin lesions in children)

Treponema pallidum-pertenue
        Yaws
        (papillomatous skin lesions in children)

ZOONOTIC SPIROCHETES

Leptospira interrogans (Zoonotic)
        Leptospirosis
        Weil syndrome

VECTOR-BORNE SPIROCHETES

Borrelia burgdorferi (Vector-borne)
        Lyme disease

Borrelia recurrentis (Vector-borne)
        Relapsing fever

Treponema pallidum

MICROAEROPHILIC

EXTRACELLULAR

FEATURES:
- **Spirochetes** : thin, tightly coiled **spiral** rods.
- Colonies: **NEVER**.

MOTILITY:
Rotates
via fibrils at
both ends

CAPSULE & GLYCOCALYX:

Complex membrane structure

EXOTOXINS:
None

_____

ENDOTOXIN:
- **Lipopolysaccharide** (LPS).

CLINICAL: (**Note**: less than **10** treponemal spirochetes can cause disease.)
- **Primary Syphilis**:
  - Symptoms: indolent (**painless**) **chancre** forms at the site of entry of *T. pallidum* (external genitalia, oral, anal, and cervix sites). Chancre starts as red, indurated (hard), **papule** then **ulcerates**. Incubation is about 3 weeks before symptoms begin. Symptoms last about 4-6 weeks; chancre heals **without scar**.
  - Syphilis is **contagious** during the **primary** stage.
  - *T. pallidum* can be isolated from the chancre.
- **Secondary Syphilis**:
  - Symptoms: **maculo-papular**, centripetal **rash** develops first on **trunk**, then spreads centrifugally to **palms**, **soles**, genitalia, and **mucus membranes** due to post-chancre **spirochetemia**. Constitutional symptoms: fever, **sore throat**, and general **lymphadenopathy** (especially epitrochlear nodes). *T. pallidum* invade **any organ** (hence **"the great pretender"**) Symptoms begin about 3 weeks to 3 months after untreated chancre is resolved, and may last 2 weeks to many months.
  - Secondary Syphilis is **contagious**.
  - *T. pallidum* can be isolated from the muco-cutaneous rash.
- **Latent syphilis**: No symptoms, but POS serological tests for *T. pallidum*
- **Secondary Syphilis Relapse**: 2° disease becomes active from latent stage. Usually occurs within 2 years of latency. **Condyloma Latum** occur.
- **Tertiary Syphilis**: ("Late Syphilis," "**lues**," or "luetic disease"):
  - Late manifestation of disease; may occur upto 40 years after latency. **Not contagious**: *T. pallidum* found in **CSF** only.
  - May affect any organ: **Neurosyphilis**: tabes dorsalis, Argyll Robertson pupil, seizures, etc. **Cardiovascular**: ascending-aorta **Aneurysm**, obliterated vaso vasorum. **Gumma** formation in bones, mucocutaneous sites, or anywhere; benign.
- **Congenital Syphilis**:
  - **Transplacental** transmission from mother (1°, 2°, or latent syphilis) to **fetus**. May lead to fetal death or newborn disease such as blindness, CNS problems, deafness, "saddle nose," "saber shins," skin rash, etc.
  - **Warning**: child is extremely **infectious at birth**.

SOURCE & TRANSMISSION:
- Horizontal transmission occurs via **sexual contact**.
- **Vertical** transmission via **transplacental** route **in utero**.
- Horizontal transmission may also occur via **blood transfusions** or direct contact with infected tissue or **contaminated fomites**.

VIRULENCE FACTORS:
- **Endotoxin**.
- Outer membrane enhances **adherence**.
- **Enzymes**: **Hyaluronidase** mediates perivascular invasion.

TREATMENT:
- **Benzathine Penicillin** for early syphilis and for prophylaxis.
- **Penicillin G** for late syphilis, congenital syphilis, and neurosyphilis.
- **Penicillin desensitization** is necessary to treat syphilis in **penicillin-allergic** patient during **pregnancy**.
- **Sexual partner** must be treated.

VACCINE & TOXOID:

None

HOST DEFENSE & IMMUNITY:
- **Plasma cells** accumulate in chancre formation.
- **IgM and IgG antibodies** develop, especially during secondary syphilis, to provide some humoral immunity.
- **T-cell** mediated immunity is important in gumma formation.
- Prolonged infection confers only **partial** immunity.

LAB TESTS:
- **Microscopy**:
spirochetes seen in skin specimen:
  Darkfield
  Immunofluorescent
- **Non-Treponemal blood tests**:
Become POS upon infection, but titers decrease during recovery.
POS indicates active disease.
  RPR (ART)
  VDRL
- **Treponemal blood tests**:
Become POS upon infection, and remain POS for patient's lifetime.
POS indicates past infection.
  FTA-abs
  MHA-TP (TPHA)

Treponema pallidum-endemicum

MICROAEROPHILIC

EXTRACELLULAR

FEATURES:
- **Spirochetes** : thin, tightly coiled **spiral** rods.
- Colonies: **NEVER**.

MOTILITY:
Rotates
via fibrils at
both ends

CAPSULE & GLYCOCALYX:
Complex membrane structure

EXOTOXINS:
None

ENDOTOXIN:
- **Lipopolysaccharide** (LPS).

CLINICAL:
- **Bejel**: (Endemic Syphilis):
  - **Primary**:
    Oral lesions; quickly resolve.
  - **Secondary**:
    Oral papules, mucosal lesions, condyloma lata.
  - **Latent**: asymptomatic.
  - **Late**:
    Gummas of bone, skin, and nasopharynx.

SOURCE & TRANSMISSION:
- Horizontal transmission occurs via **direct person-to-person** contact and via **sharing of eating or drinking utensils**.
- Infection occurs only in **children** of central **Africa**, west Asia.

VIRULENCE FACTORS:
- **Endotoxin**.
- Outer membrane enhances **adherence.**
- **Enzymes: Hyaluronidase** mediates perivascular invasion.

TREATMENT:
- **Penicillin G** for patient and contacts.

VACCINE & TOXOID:

None

HOST DEFENSE & IMMUNITY:
- **IgM and IgG antibodies** develop to provide some humoral immunity.
- **T-cell** mediated immunity is important in gumma formation.
- Prolonged infection confers only **partial** immunity.

LAB TESTS:
- **Microscopy:**
spirochetes seen in skin specimen:
    Darkfield
    Immunofluorescent
- **Non-Treponemal blood tests:**
Become POS upon infection, but titers decrease during recovery.
POS indicates active disease.
    RPR (ART)
    VDRL
- **Treponemal blood tests:**
Become POS upon infection, and remain POS for patient's lifetime.
POS indicates past infection.
    FTA-abs
    MHA-TP (TPHA)

Treponema carateum

MICROAEROPHILIC

EXTRACELLULAR

FEATURES:
- **Spirochetes** : thin, tightly coiled **spiral** rods.
- Colonies: **NEVER**.

MOTILITY:
Rotates via fibrils at both ends

CAPSULE & GLYCOCALYX:
Complex membrane structure

EXOTOXINS:
None

ENDOTOXIN:
- **Lipopolysaccharide** (LPS).

CLINICAL:
- **Pinta:** (Cutaneous treponematosis)
  - **Primary:**
    Cutaneous **pruritic papules** develop, enlarge, and coalesce.
    Incubation is about 2 weeks; symptoms last months or years; may resolve with residual permanent **hypopigmentation**.
  - **Secondary:**
    Pintids (small cutaneous scaly papules) develop at the same sites as primary lesions. Pintids may become **dyschromic** blue, brown, or gray.
    Symptoms begin about 3 months to 10 years after untreated primary lesions are resolved.
  - **Latent:** asymptomatic.
  - **Late:**
    Permanent **achromic** (de-pigmented) **macular** lesions develop at elbows, ankles, and wrists.

Note: Pinta is disfiguring, but does not shorten life span.

SOURCE & TRANSMISSION:
- Horizontal transmission occurs via **direct person-to-person** contact.
- Infection occurs only in **children** of rural **Central America, Mexico** and **South America**.

VIRULENCE FACTORS:
- **Endotoxin.**
- Outer membrane enhances **adherence.**
- **Enzymes: Hyaluronidase** mediates perivascular invasion.

TREATMENT:
- **Penicillin G** for patient and contacts.
- **Tetracycline** in penicillin allergy.

VACCINE & TOXOID:

None

HOST DEFENSE & IMMUNITY:
- **IgM and IgG antibodies** develop to provide some humoral immunity.
- **T-cell** mediated immunity is important
- Prolonged infection confers only **partial** immunity.

LAB TESTS:
- **Microscopy:**
spirochetes seen in skin specimen:
  Darkfield
  Immunofluorescent
- **Non-Treponemal blood tests:**
Become POS upon **2° lesions**, titers decrease during recovery.
POS indicates active disease.
  RPR (ART)
  VDRL
- **Treponemal blood tests:**
Become POS upon 2° lesions, and remain POS for patient's lifetime.
POS indicates past infection.
  FTA-abs
  MHA-TP (TPHA)

Treponema pallidum-pertenue

MICROAEROPHILIC

EXTRACELLULAR

FEATURES:
- **Spirochetes** : thin, tightly coiled **spiral** rods.
- Colonies: **NEVER**.

MOTILITY:
Rotates via fibrils at both ends

CAPSULE & GLYCOCALYX:
Complex membrane structure

EXOTOXINS:
None

ENDOTOXIN:
- **Lipopolysaccharide** (LPS).

CLINICAL:
- **Yaws:** (Papillomatous treponematosis)
  - **Primary:**
    Cutaneous papules develop on **extremities** then enlarge to become **papillomatous** nodules.
    Incubation is about 4 weeks; symptoms resolve in 6 months.
  - **Secondary:**
    Widespread development of **papillomatous** nodules.
    Symptoms begin weeks or months after untreated primary lesions are resolved. 2° lesions may resolve in months.
  - **Latent:** asymptomatic.
  - **Secondary Relapse:**
    Multiple relapses of 2° lesions may occur over many years.
  - **Late:**
    Cutaneous nodules and ulcers; hyperkeratosis of palms and soles; and **gummas** of bone, skin, and nasopharynx.

SOURCE & TRANSMISSION:
- Horizontal transmission occurs via **direct person-to-person** contact.
- Infection occurs only in **children** of rural **tropical** areas around the world.

VIRULENCE FACTORS:
- **Endotoxin.**
- Outer membrane enhances **adherence.**
- **Enzymes: Hyaluronidase** mediates perivascular invasion.

TREATMENT:
- **Penicillin G** for patient and contacts.
- **Tetracycline** in penicillin allergy.

VACCINE & TOXOID:

None

HOST DEFENSE & IMMUNITY:
- **IgM and IgG antibodies** develop to provide some humoral immunity.
- **T-cell** mediated immunity is important in gumma formation.
- Prolonged infection confers only **partial** immunity.

LAB TESTS:
- **Microscopy:**
spirochetes seen in skin specimen:
  Darkfield
  Immunofluorescent
- **Non-Treponemal blood tests:**
Become POS upon infection, but titers decrease during recovery.
POS indicates active disease.
  RPR (ART)
  VDRL
- **Treponemal blood tests:**
Become POS upon infection, but remain POS for patient's lifetime.
POS indicates past infection.
  FTA-abs
  MHA-TP (TPHA)

Leptospira interrogans

Zoonotic

OBLIGATE AEROBE

EXTRACELLULAR

FEATURES:
● **Spirochetes**: thin, tightly coiled **spiral** rods with **hooked ends**. "Interrogans" = question mark shape

MOTILITY:
Flagella one at each end

CAPSULE & GLYCOCALYX:
Complex membrane structure

EXOTOXINS:
None

ENDOTOXIN:
●Lipopolysaccharide (LPS).

CLINICAL:
●**Leptospirosis**: (Anicteric):
  ▪Symptoms: **Biphasic**:
  First phase (**septic phase**) occurs due to widespread dissemination with **constitutional** symptoms such as **fever**, chills, headache and myalgia.
  Incubation is about 1 week then first phase lasts about 1 week.
  An **asymptomatic period** of 2-3 days intervenes.
  Second phase (**immune phase**) occurs due to circulating antibody and **meningitis** with severe **headache**, nausea, vomiting, and myalgia.
  Symptoms of second phase last for a few days.
●**Weil Syndrome**: (Icteric):
  ▪Symptoms: **severe** form of leptospirosis, with a similar progression. Hepatic and renal dysfunction lead to **jaundice** and **renal failure**. **Myocarditis** and **cardiogenic shock** may occur. Can be **fatal**.

SOURCE & TRANSMISSION:
●**Animal kidneys** are reservoirs for *L. interrogans*, so **zoonotic transmission** occurs via contact with **animal urine**.
●Wild or domestic animals, especially **dogs**, carry *L. interrogans*
●*L. interrogans* may survive for weeks or months in streams, ponds, and moist soil contaminated by wild or domestic animals.
●Abattoir workers, farmers, veterinarians, backpackers, hunters are at risk.

VIRULENCE FACTORS:
●**Endotoxin**.
●*L. interrogans* has the ability to **penetrate mucus membranes**.
●*L. interrogans* also has the ability to **multiply very rapidly**.
●Great antigenic variation has produced well **over 200 serotypes**.
●**Enzymes: Hyaluronidase** mediates invasion.

TREATMENT:
●**Penicillin G** for patient and contacts.
●**Doxycycline** in penicillin allergy, and for prophylaxis.

VACCINE & TOXOID:
Vaccine for **animals** only.

HOST DEFENSE & IMMUNITY:
●**IgM and IgG antibodies** develop to provide some humoral immunity.
●**Immune complex deposition** may be involved in the disease process.

LAB TESTS:
●**Serologic tests**.
●**Cultures**:
Blood and **CSF**:
take specimen between 3 and 10 days after infection.
Urine:
take specimen between 1 week and 1 month after infection.

Borrelia burgdorferi

Vectors

AEROBIC

EXTRACELLULAR

FEATURES:
● **Spirochetes** : long loosely coiled **spiral** rods.
● Colonies: slow on special media.

MOTILITY:
many
Flagella

CAPSULE & GLYCOCALYX:
Complex membrane structure

EXOTOXINS:
None

_____

ENDOTOXIN:
● **Lipopolysaccharide** (LPS).

CLINICAL:
● **Lyme Disease:**
  ▪ **Stage One: Erythema Chronicum Migrans**:
      Red macule occurs at the tick bite site, this expands to become
      an **annular rash** (sometimes multiple) with **central clearing**
      (the center of the rash heals as the rash grows in diameter).
      The rash progresses to large diameter with raised **red border**.
      The rash is **painless** and **not infectious**.
      B. burgdorferi **may be cultured from biopsy of the rash**.
      Incubation is about 2 weeks; symptoms resolve in 1-2 months.
  ▪ **Stage Two:** (Neurologic and Cardiac):
      Neurologic: meningitis, encephalitis, Bell's palsy (CN VII),
      peripheral neuropathy, etc.
      Cardiac: transient A-V block. **Eyes:** conjunctivitis
      Symptoms begin weeks or months after beginning stage one.
      Stage 2 lesions may resolve in months, years or never.
  ▪ **Latent:** asymptomatic.
  ▪ **Stage Three (Late): migratory arthritis**; **chronic neurologic**; and
      musculoskeletal: intermittent and migratory arthritis, joint pain
      and swelling of the **large joints**, especially the knees.
      CNS: encephalitis; altered sensorium, memory and speech
      Symptoms begin 2 months to 2 years after beginning stage one.
      Late stage symptoms may resolve in months, years or never.
● **Congenital Lyme Disease:**
  ▪ **Very rare** transplacental transmission may occur in utero.
  ▪ May be **fatal** for neonate.

SOURCE & TRANSMISSION:
● **White-foot mouse**, **whitetail deer** and *Ixodes* **ticks** are
reservoirs for *B. burgdorferi*; **vector transmission** occurs
during **tick bite** (tick must remain attached for **24 hours** or
longer).
(horizontal transmission from tick to tick occurs.)
● **Lyme disease** is the **most common vector-borne disease** in
the **USA**, it occurs world wide.

VIRULENCE FACTORS:
● **Endotoxin**
● *B. burgdorferi* has the ability to survive in human blood and in ticks.
● *B. burgdorferi* has the ability to **resist phagocytosis.**
● *B. burgdorferi* has the ability to **adhere** to and **penetrate** epithelial cells.
● *B. burgdorferi* has the ability to **sequester** itself in joints, skin and CNS,
      thus enabling **relapses** in spite of treatment.

TREATMENT:
● **Doxycycline**
● **Amoxicillin** for children and during
pregnancy.
● **Erythromycin** for children with
penicillin allergy
● **IV Ceftriaxone** for neurologic or
cardiac symptoms.

VACCINE & TOXOID:

None

HOST DEFENSE & IMMUNITY:
● **IgM and IgG antibodies** develop against
various spirochete components.
● **Classic complement** pathway aids in
opsonization.
● **T-cell** mediated **delayed hypersensitivity**
and **immune-complex** deposition may have
role in joint inflammation.

LAB TESTS:
● **Serologic tests**.
● **Cultures:**
Biopsy of stage one rash only.

Borrelia recurrentis

Vectors

AEROBIC

EXTRACELLULAR

FEATURES:
- **Spirochetes** : long loosely coiled **spiral** rods.
- Colonies: slow on special media.

MOTILITY:
many
Flagella

CAPSULE & GLYCOCALYX:
Complex membrane structure

EXOTOXINS:
None

ENDOTOXIN:
- **Lipopolysaccharide** (LPS).

CLINICAL:
- **Relapsing Fever:**
  - **First Febrile Attack:**
    - Lice get **crushed** on skin, the *B. recurrentis* spirochetes get released then **penetrate** through epithelium to invade the **blood stream**.
  - Symptoms: **high fever**, chills, headache, myalgia and splenomegaly. Incubation is about 1 week then first attack lasts about 1 week.
  - **Latent:** antibodies effectively clear spirochetes from the bloodstream, but some survive by sequestration in various organs, especially the spleen and liver. Patient becomes **afebrile** during latency. Latency lasts about 1 week.
  - **Relapse:** symptoms return for a few days as the surface antigens get changed to enable *B. recurrentis* to evade antibodies, thus a second spirochetemia ensues to cause fever.
  - **Latent:** a second asymptomatic interval intervenes
  - **Relapse:** symptoms return again. 2 or 3 relapses are common.

Note: Infection may be **fatal**, usually due to hypotension and **shock** during the first febrile attack.

SOURCE & TRANSMISSION:
- **Humans** are reservoir for *B. recurrentis*; **vector transmission** occurs during **human lice being crushed** on mucus membranes or skin; the spirochetes then penetrate the epithelium and travel in the blood. Transmission is **not** via lice bites or feces.
- **Relapsing fever** occurs world wide.

VIRULENCE FACTORS:
- **Endotoxin**
- **Variable Major Protein:**
  - Surface antigen protein may be **varied** many times throughout the course of infection. This enables *B. recurrentis* to escape opsonization by antibody and complement, thus **relapses** occur.
- *B. recurrentis* has the ability to survive in human blood and lice lymph.
- *B. recurrentis* has the ability to **resist phagocytosis.**
- *B. recurrentis* has the ability to **adhere** to and **penetrate** epithelial cells.
- *B. recurrentis* has the ability to **sequester** itself in internal organs during afebrile periods, thus enabling **relapses**.

TREATMENT:
- **Doxycycline**
- **Erythromycin** for children and during pregnancy.

VACCINE & TOXOID:
None

HOST DEFENSE & IMMUNITY:
- **IgM and IgG antibodies** develop against various spirochete surface antigens, but the ability of *B. recurrentis* to vary its antigens make antibodies ultimately ineffective.
- **Cytokines** play an important role.

LAB TESTS:
- **Peripheral blood smear:**
Dark-field microscopy, giemsa stain, or wright stain.

Chapter 13

CHLAMYDIA

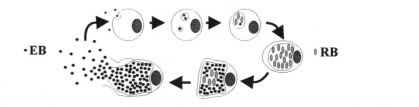

·EB **·RB**

RESPIRATORY DISEASE

Chlamydia pneumoniae
    Atypical pneumonia
    Bronchitis

ZOONOTIC CHLAMYDIA

Chlamydia psittaci (Zoonotic)
    Atypical pneumonia

SEXUALLY TRANSMITTED DISEASE

Chlamydia trachomatis
    Sexually transmitted diseases
        Urethritis
        Proctitis
        Cervicitis
        PID
        Lymphogranuloma Venereum
    Trachoma (eye infection)
    Neonatal infections
    Reiter syndrome

Chlamydia pneumoniae

GRAM STAIN:
Null
(stain poorly)
No Peptidoglycan

OBLIGATE ANAEROBE

RB = OBLIGATE INTRACELLULAR

EB = EXTRACELLULAR

FEATURES:
- Biphasic:
Infectious Extracellular form:
    Elemental Bodies (EB)
        "Pear shaped"
Obligate Intracellular form:
    Reticulate Bodies (RB).
- Colonies: require **cell culture**.

MOTILITY:
None

CAPSULE & GLYCOCALYX:
None

EXOTOXINS:
None.

ENDOTOXIN:
- **Lipopolysaccharide** (LPS): similar to Gram NEG bacteria.

CLINICAL:
- **Pneumonia: Atypical Pneumonia**.
  - Respiratory infection by *C. pneumoniae* is very common.
  Infection is usually mild or asymptomatic, but can be **fatal**.
  - Symptomatic infection occurs most often in the **elderly**.
  - **Chest X-ray** usually shows unilateral, lower lobe involvement.
  - Symptoms: **interstitial pneumonia** with **non-productive cough** and
  inspiratory crackles, **fever**, chills, headache, and chest pain.
  - Symptoms begin gradually over days to weeks.
  - Symptoms may last for weeks or months, and **relapses** may occur.
- **Bronchitis**.

SOURCE & TRANSMISSION:
- **Humans** are the only reservoirs for *C. pneumoniae*.
- Horizontal transmission occurs via **respiratory droplets**.
- **Epidemics** can occur.

VIRULENCE FACTORS:
- **Unique life cycle:**
  Elementary Bodies (EB=300 nm) enter host cells via several
  mechanisms; EBs organize as **Reticulate Bodies** (RB=1000nm)
  which replicate to produce new Elemental Bodies; the host cell
  ruptures to release the EBs so the cycle can continue.
- *Chlamydia pneumoniae* survive in Macros or epithelial cells;
  but are killed in PMNs.
- *Chlamydia pneumoniae* have the ability to cause **recurrent** or **persistent**
  infections which often lead to greater tissue damage and scarring
  than the initial infection.

TREATMENT:
- **Doxycycline**.
- **Erythromycin**
For children and pregnant women.

VACCINE & TOXOID:
None

HOST DEFENSE & IMMUNITY:
- **PMNs** are the most effective defense.
- **T-cells**, Macros, eosinophils and plasma
cells are all activated.
- **Cytokines** are effective.
- **Previous infection** confers **no protective
immunity** against subsequent infection.

LAB TESTS:
- PCR may be useful.
- Few tests, if any, are helpful.

Chlamydia psittaci

GRAM STAIN:
Null
(stain poorly)
No Peptidoglycan

Zoonotic

OBLIGATE ANAEROBE

RB = OBLIGATE INTRACELLULAR

EB = EXTRACELLULAR

FEATURES:
●Biphasic:
Infectious Extracellular form:
        Elemental Bodies (EB)
Obligate Intracellular form:
        Reticulate Bodies (RB).
●Colonies: require **cell culture**.

MOTILITY:
None

CAPSULE & GLYCOCALYX:
None

EXOTOXINS:
None.

ENDOTOXIN:
●**Lipopolysaccharide** (LPS): similar to Gram NEG bacteria.

CLINICAL:
●**Pneumonia: Atypical Pneumonia**.
    ▪Infection is usually mild or asymptomatic, but can be **fatal**.
    ▪Symptomatic infection occurs most often in the **elderly**.
    ▪**Chest X-ray** usually shows unilateral, lower lobe involvement.
    ▪Symptoms: **interstitial pneumonia** with **non-productive cough** and
        inspiratory crackles, **fever**, chills, headache, and chest pain.
    ▪Incubation is about 1-2 weeks
    ▪Symptoms may last for weeks or months, and **relapses** may occur.
●*C. psittaci* spread to the RES and cause **hepatosplenomegaly** with **jaundice**.
●*C. psittaci* **disseminate** then via **hematogenous** route to:
    ▪**CNS:** encephalitis, seizures, and coma, can be **fatal**.
    ▪**Heart:** pericarditis, myocarditis, and endocarditis; can be **fatal**.
    ▪**GI Tract:** nausea, vomiting, and diarrhea.
    ▪**Thyroid:** thyrotoxicosis.
    ▪*C. psittaci* complications can affect any organ.

SOURCE & TRANSMISSION:
●**Birds** and **poultry** are reservoirs for *C. psittaci*, so
zoonotic transmission occurs via **contact** with birds and poultry
●Transmission from bird to bird, or to bird offspring, is how the
reservoir population of *C. psittaci* is maintained
●**Abatoir** workers, **veterinarians**, **farmers**, **pet shop** owners,
zoo keepers, or anyone in contact with an infected bird is at risk.

VIRULENCE FACTORS:
●**Unique life cycle:**
        Elementary Bodies (EB=300 nm) enter host cells via several
        mechanisms; EBs organize as **Reticulate Bodies** (RB=1000nm)
        which replicate to produce new Elemental Bodies; the host cell
        ruptures to release the EBs so the cycle can continue.
●*Chlamydia psittaci* survive in Macros or epithelial cells;
        but are killed in PMNs.
●*Chlamydia psittaci* has the ability to cause **recurrent** or **persistent**
        infections which often lead to greater tissue damage and scarring
        than the initial infection.

TREATMENT:
●**Doxycycline**.
●**Erythromycin**
For children and pregnant women.
●**Prevention:**
Prophylactic Doxycycline for birds.

VACCINE & TOXOID:
None

HOST DEFENSE & IMMUNITY:
●**PMNs** are the most effective defense.
●**T-cells**, Macros, eosinophils and plasma
cells are all activated.
●**Cytokines** are effective.
●**Previous infection** confers **no protective
immunity** against subsequent infection.

LAB TESTS:
●**Serology** tests for high titer of
complement-fixing antibodies
may be useful for diagnosis, but it
is not species-specific.
●**Cell-culture** may be done, but it
is dangerous.

Chlamydia trachomatis

GRAM STAIN:

Null
(stain poorly)
No Peptidoglycan

OBLIGATE ANAEROBE

RB = OBLIGATE INTRACELLULAR

EB = EXTRACELLULAR

FEATURES:
- Biphasic:
Infectious Extracellular form:
    Elemental Bodies (EB)
Obligate Intracellular form:
    Reticulate Bodies (RB).
- Colonies: require **cell culture**.

MOTILITY:

None

CAPSULE & GLYCOCALYX:

None

EXOTOXINS:
None.

ENDOTOXIN:
- **Lipopolysaccharide** (LPS): similar to Gram NEG bacteria.

CLINICAL:
- **NOTE:** *Chlamydia trachomatis* is the **#1 cause of STD in the USA**.
- **Male STD:**
  - **Urethritis, Epididymitis:**
        Symptoms: **urethral discharge**, dysuria, and **hemospermia**.
        Most often **asymptomatic** in men.
  - **Proctitis:** in homosexual men from anal intercourse.
- **Female STD:**
  - **Cervicitis, endometritis, salpingitis**, and **PID**:
        Symptoms: **vaginal discharge**, dysuria, pain, bleeding.
        Often **asymptomatic** in women. May cause **sterility**.
  - **Proctitis:** from anal intercourse.
- **Lymphogranyuloma Venereum STD:**
  - Incubation is about 2 weeks, but **females** often remain **asymptomatic**.
  - Stage one: Genital/anal papule arises at site of infection; heals rapidly.
  - Stage two: **Inguinal lymphadenopathy - "buboes"** - arise along with
        constitutional symptoms such as fever, headache, myalgia.
        May present as **proctitis** due to anal intercourse.
  - Symptoms may spontaneously resolve or become a chronic condition.
- **Trachoma:**
  - **Chronic inflammation of eye** due to hand-eye **autoinoculation**.
  - Often leads to **blindness**, does not occur as a neonatal infection.
- **Neonatal infections:** (Due to passage through infected vagina)
  - **Inclusion Conjunctivitis:** arises 1-2 weeks after birth; no blindness.
  - **Infant Atypical Pneumonia:** arises 5-25 weeks after birth.
- Post-*Chlamydia* **Reiter Syndrome**:
  - Arthritic disease associated with HLA-B27 genotype.

SOURCE & TRANSMISSION:
- Humans are the only reservoir of *Chlamydia trachomatis*
- Transmission is via **sexual contact** or autoinoculation of the
infection to other parts of the body.
- **Vertical transmission** from mother to neonate **during birth**,
by passage through infected vagina.

VIRULENCE FACTORS:
- **Unique life cycle:**
      Elementary Bodies (EB=300 nm) enter host cells via several
      mechanisms; EBs organize as **Reticulate Bodies** (RB=1000nm)
      which replicate to produce new Elemental Bodies; the host cell
      ruptures to release the EBs so the cycle can continue.
- *Chlamydia trachomatis* survive in Macros or epithelial cells;
      but are killed in PMNs.
- *Chlamydia trachomatis* has the ability to cause **recurrent** or **persistent**
      infections which often lead to greater tissue damage and scarring
      than the initial infection.

TREATMENT:
- **Doxycycline**.
- **Erythromycin**
For children and pregnant women.
- **Cefoxitin** plus **Doxycycline** when
concurrent *N. gonorrhea* infection.
- Lymphogranuloma venereum:
Requires **aspiration** of lymph nodes.
- **Sexual partner** must be treated.
- **Condoms** and **sex education** for
prevention.

VACCINE & TOXOID:

None

HOST DEFENSE & IMMUNITY:
- **PMNs** are the most effective defense.
- **T-cells**, Macros, eosinophils and plasma
cells are all activated.
- **Cytokines** are effective.
- **Previous infection** confers **no protective
immunity** against subsequent infection.

LAB TESTS:
- **Specimens:** are obtained from female
endocervical cytobrushing; male
urethral swabbing; or scraping of
infected conjunctiva.
- Direct **immunofluorescent**, Iodine,
ELISA or Giemsa stained smears show
triangular-shape intra-cytoplasmic
inclusion bodies (the **RBs**).
- Direct **immunofluorescent** or ELISA
staining of specimen may reveal **EBs**.
- Prior to testing, specimens may be
cultured by **cell-culture** techniques, for
greater specificity.
- DNA probe and PCR amplification or
EIA from **Urine** specimen.
- Serological tests are not helpful.

Chapter 14

MYCOPLASMA AND UREAPLASMA

SEXUALLY TRANSMITTED DISEASE

Mycoplasma hominis
        Sexually transmitted diseases
           UTI
           PID
      Perinatal
           Post-partum fever
           Post-abortion fever

RESPIRATORY DISEASE

Mycoplasma pneumoniae
        Atypical pneumonia
        Bronchitis

UREAPLASMA SEXUALLY TRANSMITTED DISEASE

Ureaplasma urealyticum
        Sexually transmitted diseases
           Urethritis
      Perinatal
           Low birthweight newborns
           Chorioamnionitis

Mycoplasma hominis

GRAM STAIN:
Null
(stain poorly)
No Cell Wall

AEROBIC

EXTRACELLULAR

FEATURES:
●**Smallest free-living organisms**.
Pliable membrane contains **sterols**,
and **no cell wall**.
●Colonies: **extracellular** growth
on agar media yields **microscopic**
characteristic"**fried egg**"colonies.
Intracellular growth on cell

MOTILITY:
None

CAPSULE & GLYCOCALYX:
None

EXOTOXINS:
None

ENDOTOXIN:
None

CLINICAL:
●**UTI: Acute Pyelonephritis**
 ▪Symptoms: flank pain, fever, dysuria.
 ▪May progress to PID
●**Perinatal Infection:**
 ▪**Post-Partum Fever and Post-Abortion Fever:**
 Fever will last a few days following birth or following abortion.

SOURCE & TRANSMISSION:
●**Humans** are the only reservoirs for **M. hominis**.
●Horizontal transmission occurs via **sexual contact**.
●Temporary colonization of neonates may occur by passage
through infected vagina during birth; usually inconsequential.

VIRULENCE FACTORS:
●**Antimicrobial Resistance:**
 ▪Lack of cell wall foils drugs that target cell wall components.
●**Hydrogen Peroxide Production:**
 ▪May contribute to mucosal damage.
●**M. hominis** has the ability to survive intracellularly, but is does
 most damage to host cells at extracellular locations.
●**Special Nutrient Requirements:**
 ▪**Cholesterol**, nucleic acid precursors, amino acids, etc.
●**Sterol Cytoplasmic Membrane:**
 ▪Unique feature of *Mycoplasmataceae* family.

TREATMENT:
●**Doxycycline**
●**Erythromycin**
For children and pregnant women;
also for doxycycline-resistant strains.

VACCINE & TOXOID:
None

HOST DEFENSE & IMMUNITY:
●**Antibodies** and **T-cells** are important.
●**Previous infection** confers **no protective
immunity** against subsequent infection.

LAB TESTS:
●**Culture:**
 From genitourinary tract.
 Grows in 1-2 weeks.
●Glucose fermentation   NEG
●Metabolizes **Arginine**.

Mycoplasma pneumoniae

GRAM STAIN:
Null
(stain poorly)
No Cell Wall

AEROBIC

EXTRACELLULAR

FEATURES:
●**Smallest free-living organisms**.
Pliable membrane contains **sterols**,
and **no cell wall**.
●Colonies: **extracellular** growth
on agar media yields **microscopic**
characteristic"**mulberry**"colonies.
Intracellular growth on cell

MOTILITY:

None

CAPSULE & GLYCOCALYX:

None

EXOTOXINS:
None

ENDOTOXIN:
None

CLINICAL:
●Pneumonia: Atypical Pneumonia.
▪*M. pneumoniae* is the **most common cause of Atypical pneumonia**.
Infection is usually mild or asymptomatic, but can be **fatal**.
▪Infection occurs most often in teenagers and young adults.
especially **college students** and **military troops**.
▪**Chest X-ray** usually shows unilateral, lower lobe involvement.
▪Symptoms: **interstitial pneumonia** with **non-productive cough** and
inspiratory crackles, **fever**, chills, headache, and chest pain.
▪Incubation is 2-3 weeks.
▪Symptoms may last for weeks or months, and **relapses** may occur.
▪**Complications:**
Raynauds phenomena may occur in *M. pneumonia* infection
due to **cold-agglutinin antibodies**, this can lead to necrosis of
fingers and toes if it occurs in **Sickle cell anemia** patients.
●**Bronchitis.**

SOURCE & TRANSMISSION:
●**Humans** are the only reservoirs for *M. pneumoniae*.
●**Horizontal transmission occurs via **respiratory droplets**
mostly among **college students** and **military** troops worldwide.
●**Epidemics** can occur.

VIRULENCE FACTORS:
●**Antimicrobial Resistance:**
▪Lack of cell wall foils drugs that target cell wall components.
●**Adhesin Protein P1:**
▪Enables attachment to epithelial cells, especially ciliated cells.
●**Hydrogen Peroxide Production:**
▪May contribute to mucosal damage.
●*M. pneumonia* has the ability to survive intracellularly, but does
most damage to host cells at extracellular locations.
●**Special Nutrient Requirements:**
▪**Cholesterol**, nucleic acid precursors, amino acids, etc.
●**Sterol Cytoplasmic Membrane:**
▪Unique feature of *Mycoplasmataceae* family.

TREATMENT:
●**Doxycycline**
●**Erythromycin**
For children and pregnant women.

VACCINE & TOXOID:

None

HOST DEFENSE & IMMUNITY:
●**Antibodies** and **T-cells** are important.
●**Autoantibodies are produced:**
Several autoagglutinins, especially
IgM Cold Isohemagglutinins
●**Cytokines** are activated, except IL-2.
●**Previous infection** confers **no protective
immunity** against subsequent infection.

LAB TESTS:
●**Culture:**
Of sputum; takes weeks.
●**Gram Stain** of sputum to rule
out other causative organisms.
●**Cold Agglutinins   POS**
(special RBC IgM blood test)
●**Glucose fermentation   POS**
●**Tetrazolium Dye reduction:**
Blue to Yellow.

Ureaplasma urealyticum

GRAM STAIN:
Null
(stain poorly)
No Cell Wall

AEROBIC

EXTRACELLULAR

FEATURES:
●**Smallest free-living organisms**.
Pliable membrane contains **sterols**,
and **no cell wall**.
●Colonies: **extracellular** growth
on agar media yields **microscopic**
characteristic "fried egg" colonies.
Intracellular growth on cell

MOTILITY:

None

CAPSULE & GLYCOCALYX:

None

EXOTOXINS:
None

ENDOTOXIN:
None

CLINICAL:
●**Urethritis:** does not progress to PID.
●**Perinatal Infection:**
  ▪**Low Birth-Weight Newborns**.
  ▪Chorioamnionitis: rare.

SOURCE & TRANSMISSION:
●**Humans** are the only reservoirs for **U. urealyticum**.
●Horizontal transmission occurs via **sexual contact**.
●Temporary colonization of neonates may occur by passage
through infected vagina during birth; usually inconsequential.

VIRULENCE FACTORS:
●**Antimicrobial Resistance:**
  ▪Lack of cell wall foils drugs that target cell wall components.
●**U. urealyticum** has the ability to survive intracellularly, but is does
    most damage to host cells at extracellular locations.
●**Special Nutrient Requirements:**
  ▪**Cholesterol**, nucleic acid precursors, amino acids, etc.
●**Sterol Cytoplasmic Membrane:**
  ▪Unique feature of *Mycoplasmataceae* family.
●**U. urealyticum** can split **urea** as an energy source.

TREATMENT:
●**Doxycycline**
●**Erythromycin**
For children and pregnant women;
also for doxycycline-resistant strains.

VACCINE & TOXOID:

None

HOST DEFENSE & IMMUNITY:
●**Antibodies** and **T-cells** are important.
●**Previous infection** confers **no protective
immunity** against subsequent infection.

LAB TESTS:
●**Culture:**
    From genitourinary tract.
    Grows within 2 days.
    Very TINY colonies.
    Requires Urea.
●Glucose fermentation   NEG

Chapter 15

BACTERIA CROSS REFERENCE (Part 1)

OBLIGATE AEROBES
Pseudomonas aeruginosa
  Mycobacterium spp
Leptospira interrogans

OBLIGATE ANAEROBES
Clostridium botulinum
Clostridium difficile
Clostridium perfringens
Clostridium tetani
Actinomyces israelii
Peptostreptococcus spp
Propionibacterium acnes
Bacteroides fragilis
Fusobacterium spp
Prevotella spp
Chlamydia spp

MICROAEROPHILIC
Helicobacter pylori
Campylobacter jejuni
Treponema spp

BIPOLAR STAINING
["Safety pin pattern" ⬤▭]
Haemophilus influenzae
Francisella tularensis
Pasteurella multocida
Yersinia pestis

OBLIGATE INTRACELLULAR
Rickettsia spp
Ehrlichia spp
Chlamydia spp

INTRACELLULAR
Listeria monocytogenes
Neisseria spp
Legionella pneumophilia
Salmonella spp
Shigella spp
Brucella spp
Coxiella burnetii
Francisella tularensis
Yersinia pestis
  Mycobacterium spp
Nocardia asteroides

UNUSUAL SHAPE BACTERIA
Corynebacterium diphtheriae
    (club; Chinese letter clumps)
Listeria monocytogenes
    (Chinese letter clumps)
Clostridium tetani
    (club or tennis racquet)
Neisseria spp (coffee bean pairs)
Helicobacter pylori ("S" or comma)
Vibrio spp ("S" or comma)
Bacillus anthracis (boxcar)
Campylobacter jejuni
    ("S"or comma)
Actinomyces spp (filamentous)
  Mycobacterium tuberculosis(cords)
Nocardia spp (filamentous)
Chlamydia spp
    (elemental/reticulate bodies)

MOTILITY
Bacillus cereus
Listeria monocytogenes (tumble)
Clostridium difficile
Clostridium tetani
Proteus spp
Morganella spp
Providencia spp
Enterobacter cloacae
Serratia marcescens
Uropathogenic E. coli
Legionella pneumophilia
Pseudomonas aeruginosa
Helicobacter pylori (cork screw)
Vibrio spp
Enteric *E. coli*
Salmonella spp
Campylobacter jejuni (darting)
Yersinia (in culture only)
Bartonella spp (twitching)
  Treponema spp(rotate)
  Leptospira interrogans
  Borrelia spp

PIGMENT PRODUCING
Corynebacterium diphtheriae
    (gray-black)
Pseudomonas aeruginosa
    (blue-green)
Serratia marcescens (red)
Prevotella melaninogenica
    (brown)
Legionella pneumophilia
    (brown)
Nontuberculous *Mycobacteria*
    (yellow)

CAPSULES
Group A Streptococcus
    (Hyaluronic acid)
Group B Streptococcus
Streptococcus pneumoniae
Neisseria spp
Moraxella catarrhalis
Bordetella pertussis
Haemophilus influenzae
Klebsiella pneumoniae
E. coli (sometimes)
Salmonella spp
Bacillus anthracis
    (polypeptide D-glutamate)
Francisella tularensis (lipid)
Pasteurella multocida
Yersinia pestis
    (protein-polysaccharide)
Bacteroides fragilis
Prevotella melaninogenica
Mycobacterium spp
    (lipid/polypeptide)

GLYCOCALYX
Staphylococcus epidermidis
Streptococcus Viridans Group
Pseudomonas aeruginosa

SPORES
Bacillus spp (spores need oxygen)
Clostridium spp (anaerobic)
Coxiella burnetii

EXOTOXIN PRODUCING
Staphylococcus aureus
Group A Streptococcus
Bacillus spp
Corynebacterium diphtheriae
Listeria monocytogenes
Clostridium spp
Uropathogenic E. coli
Bordetella pertussis
Pseudomonas aeruginosa
Vibrio spp
Entero Toxigenic E. coli
Entero Hemorrhagic E. coli
Shigella spp

IgA PROTEASE
Streptococcus pneumoniae
Neisseria spp
Haemophilus influenzae

NO CELL WALL
[Require cholesterol culture]
Mycoplasma
Ureaplasma

GRAM NULL
[Do not stain with Gram stain]
All Spirochetes
Chlamydia spp
Mycoplasma
Ureaplasma

GRAM VARIABLE
[POS or NEG with Gram stain}
Gardnerella vaginalis

FEW ORGANISMS NEEDED TO CAUSE INFECTION
Shigella spp
Coxiella burnetii
Rickettsia spp
Bartonella spp
Chlamydia spp

MANY ORGANISMS NEEDED TO CAUSE INFECTION
Salmonella spp
Vibrio spp

NO INVITRO GROWTH
Mycobacterium leprae
(grow on foot pad of living mouse)
Treponema spp

CELL CULTURE GROWTH
Coxiella burnetii
Rickettsia spp
Ehrlichia spp
Chlamydia spp

UNUSUAL CULTURES
Proteus spp (swarming, putrid)
Corynebacterium diphtheriae
    (black)
Pseudomonas aeruginosa
    (blue-green, fruity)
Mycoplasma and **Ureaplasma**
    (fried egg)
Mycoplasma pneumoniae
    (mulberry)

BACTERIA CROSS REFERENCE (Part 2): Categories Of Common Bacterial Toxins

ADP-Ribosylating Toxins
V. cholera Cholera Toxin
ETEC Cholera-like LT Toxin

C. diphtheriae Diphtheria Toxin
(Blocks host EF2)
P. aeruginosa Exotoxin A
Diphtheria-like toxin
(Blocks host EF2)

C. botulinum C2 Enterotoxin
(This in not botulism neurotoxin)
C. perfringens Iota Toxin

B. pertussis Pertussis Toxin

Adenylate Cyclase Toxins
B. pertussis
Adenylate Cyclase Toxin
(This is not pertussis toxin)
B. anthracis
Edema Factor

Toxins ⇧ Adenylate Cyclase:
⇧ cAMP:
B. pertussis
Adenylate Cyclase Toxin
(This is not pertussis toxin)
B. anthracis
Edema Factor

V. cholera Cholera Toxin
ETEC Cholera-like LT Toxin

Toxins ⇧ cGMP:
ETEC Cholera-like ST Toxin

G-Protein Mediated:
V. cholera Cholera Toxin
(Turn on the "on signal")
ETEC Cholera-like LT Toxin
(Turn on the "on signal")

B. pertussis Pertussis Toxin
(Turn off the "off signal")

Metallo Protease Toxins
C. botulinum Botulinum Toxin
C. tetani Tetanus toxin
B. anthracis Lethal Factor

Neuro Toxins:
C. botulinum Botulinum Toxin
(Flaccid paralysis)
C. tetani Tetanus toxin
(Spastic paralysis)

RNA Glycosidas Toxins
Shigella spp Shiga Toxin
(blocks 28s rRNA of 60s subunit)
EHEC Shiga-like Toxin (SLT)
(blocks 28s rRNA of 60s subunit)

Protein Synthesis Inhibition
Shigella spp Shiga Toxin
(blocks 28s rRNA of 60s subunit)
EHEC Shiga-like Toxin (SLT)
(blocks 28s rRNA of 60s subunit)

C. diphtheriae Diphtheria Toxin
(Blocks host EF2)
P. aeruginosa Exotoxin A
Diphtheria-like toxin
(Blocks host EF2)

Enterotoxins:
S. aureus Toxin A, Toxin F
B. cereus Enterotoxin
C. botulinum C2 Enterotoxin
(This in not botulism neurotoxin)
C. difficile Enterotoxin
C. perfringens Enterotoxin

V. cholera Cholera Toxin
ETEC Cholera-like LT Toxin
ETEC Cholera-like ST Toxin

V. parahaemolyticus Enterotoxin

Shigella spp Shiga Toxin
(blocks 28s rRNA of 60s subunit)
EHEC Shiga-like Toxin (SLT)
(blocks 28s rRNA of 60s subunit)

NOTE: 1. These light microscope color plates represent typical specimens(not ideal specimens) as encountered in clinical practice.
2. All of the color plates on this page are magnified to equal high power to allow meaningful comparison of relative sizes.

Bacteria Cross Reference   102

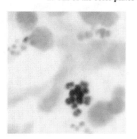

Staphylococcus aureus

Abscess (Gram stain)

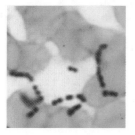

Streptococcus Group A

Blood (Gram stain)

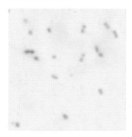

Streptococcus Group B

CSF (Gram stain)

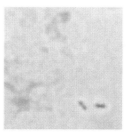

Streptococcus pneumoniae

Sputum (Gram stain)

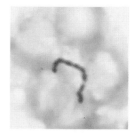

Streptococcus Group A

Blood (Gram stain)

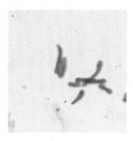

Corynebacterium diphtheriae

Culture (Gram stain)

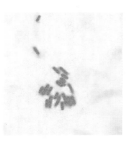

Listeria monocytogenes

Sputum (Gram stain)

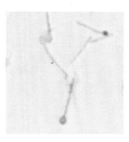

Clostridium tetani

Culture (Gram stain)

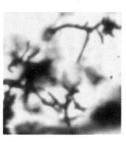

Actinomyces israelii

Brain abscess (Gram stain)

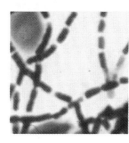

Bacillus anthracis

Tissue biopsy (Gram stain)

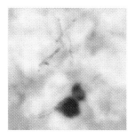

Mycobacterium tuberculosis

Sputum (Acid Fast stain)

Nocardia asteroides

Brain abscess

(Modified Acid Fast stain)

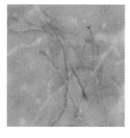

Nocardia asteroides

Brain abscess

(Gram stain)

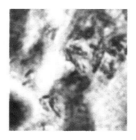

Mycobacterium leprae

Skin biopsy (Fite stain)

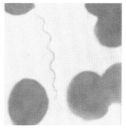

Borrelia recurrentis

Blood smear (Giemsa stain)

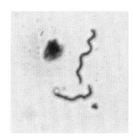

Borrelia burgdorferi

Skin biopsy (Giemsa stain)

NOTE: 1. These light microscope color plates represent typical specimens(not ideal specimens) as encountered in clinical practice.
2. All of the color plates on this page are magnified to equal high power (except as noted) to allow meaningful comparison of relative sizes.

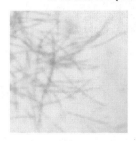

Fusobacterium spp

Abscess (Gram stain)

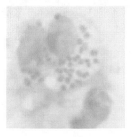

Neisseria gonorrhoeae in PMN.

Urethral discharge (Gram stain)

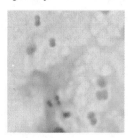

Neisseria meningitides

CSF (Gram stain)

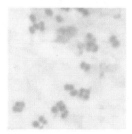

Moraxella catarrhalis

Sputum (Gram stain)

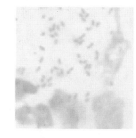

Haemophilus influenzae

Sputum (Gram stain)

Klebsiella pneumoniae

Sputum (Gram stain)

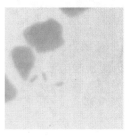

Pseudomonas aeruginosa

Sputum (Gram stain)

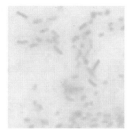

Pseudomonas aeruginosa

Sputum in Cystic Fibrosis (Gram stain)

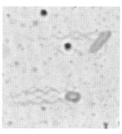

Proteus vulgaris

Urine (Flagella stain)

Helicobacter pylori

Stomach biopsy (Gram stain)

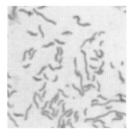

Vibrio cholera

Culture (Gram stain)

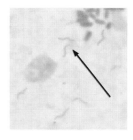

Campylobacter jejuni

Feces (Gram stain)

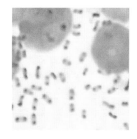

Yersinia pestis

Blood (Gram stain)

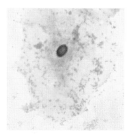

Ehrlichia chaffeensis

Blood smear (Giemsa stain)

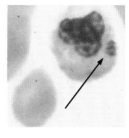

Gardneralla vaginalis Clue Cell.

Vaginal smear (Gram stain)

Medium power view

Chapter 16

DNA VIRUSES

Single-strand linear DNA
Icosahedral
No envelope

Parvovirus
    B19 virus
        Erythema Infectiosum
        Hydrops Fetalis
        Sickle cell aplastic crisis
    Dependovirus
        Asymptomatic

Double-strand linear DNA
Icosahedral
No envelope

Adenovirus
    1, 2, 3, 5 Intussusception
    3, 7 Pharyngoconjunctivitis
    3, 4, 7 Atypical pneumonia
    8, 19, 37 Keratoconjunctivitis
    11, 21 Hemorrhagic cystitis
    40, 41 Diarrhea

Double-strand Circular DNA
Icosahedral
No envelope

Papovavirus
Human Papillomavirus
    HPV-1, HPV-2 Common warts
    HPV-6, HPV-11 Genital warts
    HPV-16, HPV-18 Cervical carcinoma
Polyomavirus
    JC virus PML
    BK virus asymptomatic

Partial double-strand Circular DNA
Icosahedral
Envelope

Hepadnavirus
    Hepatitis B
        Acute Hepatitis
        Chronic Hepatitis
        Carrier State Hepatitis
        Hepatocellular carcinoma
    Hepatitis D
Single-strand circular RNA
Double envelope
Defective virus
        Acute Hepatitis
        Chronic Hepatitis
        Carrier State Hepatitis
        Hepatocellular carcinoma

Double-strand linear DNA
Icosahedral
Envelope

Herpes virus
    Alpha virus
        HSV-1 Herpes labialis
        HSV-2 Herpes genitalis
        VZV Chicken pox
            Herpes zoster
            Reye syndrome
    Beta virus
        CMV Mononucleosis
            Retinitis
            Congenital encephalitis
    Gamma virus
        EBV Mononucleosis
            Malignancy
        HHV-6 Roseola

Double-strand Linear DNA
Complex nucleocapsid
Double envelope
Pox virus
Orthopoxvirus
    Vaccinia Cow pox
    Variola Small pox
Molluscum contagiosum virus
        Genital infection

Family: PARVO VIRUS

GENERA AND SPECIES:
Parvovirus:
B19
Dependovirus:
Adeno-associated virus
Herpes-associated virus

GENOME:
ss linear DNA
+ or (-) sense.

SEGMENTATION:
No other segments

NUCLEOCAPSID:
Icosahedral

LOCATION OF REPLICATION:
Nucleus

ENVELOPE:
No Envelope

EFFECT ON HOST CELL:
Causes **host cell lysis**

SPECIAL FACTS:
- Parvoviruses are the only **single-stranded DNA viruses**; and the single strands may be **positive sense** or **negative sense** depending on strain.
- Parvoviruses are very durable, they can survive in the environment for many years and they can endure high temperatures for many hours.

Genus: Parvovirus

Species: B19 virus
- Disease:
  - **Erythema Infectiosum: "Slapped cheeks"** Red macular facial rash, limited to cheeks.
  - **Erythroid Precursor Lysis:** Destroys RBC precursors of host bone marrow; causes hemolytic anemia.
    - **-Fatal Aplastic Crisis** occurs when RBC precursors are destroyed in a patient with **sickle cell disease.**
    - **-Fatal Hemolytic Anemia** occurs when RBC precursors are destroyed in patient with prior **aplastic anemia.**
    - **-Chronic anemia** occurs when RBC precursors are destroyed in immunocompromised patient.
  - **Hydrops Fetalis:** causes **abortion** of fetus if mother gets infected during **pregnancy.**
  - Arthritis.
- Transmission:
  - **Horizontal** via **respiratory route.**
  - Horizontal via blood transfusions.
  - **Vertical** from mother to fetus via **transplacental** route
  - **Spring** season.
- Geographic Range: **World-wide.**
- Diagnosis: **Serology:**
  - B19 DNA detection indicates current infection.
  - **B19-specific IgM antibody** indicates recent infection.
  - **B19-specific IgG antibody** indicates past infection.
- Treatment:
  - Infection is most often benign and self-limited.
  - **Blood transfusion** during a severe aplastic crisis.
  - **IV immunoglobulin** for immunocompromised cases.
  - Infection must be avoided during pregnancy.
- Immunity: post-infectious immunity is long lasting.
- Vaccine: none.

Genus: Dependovirus

Species: Adeno-dependent Dependovirus
- NOTE: All Dependoviruses require **co-infection** with a **double-stranded DNA** virus in order to establish infection.
- Infection is not known to cause disease.

Species: Herpes-dependent Dependovirus
- NOTE: All Dependoviruses require **co-infection** with a **double-stranded DNA** virus in order to establish infection.
- Infection is not known to cause disease.

Family: ADENO VIRUS

GENERA AND SPECIES:	GENOME:
Adenovirus: 47 serotypes.	**DS linear DNA**

SEGMENTATION:
No other segments

NUCLEOCAPSID:
Icosahedral
with Fiber Spikes.

LOCATION OF REPLICATION:
Nucleus

ENVELOPE:
No Envelope

EFFECT ON HOST CELL:
Causes **host cell lysis**

SPECIAL FACTS:

- Adenovirus has **hemagglutinin fibers** protruding from each of the 12 vertices of the nucleocapsid; this provides serotype-specific antigens.
- **Capsid** basic structure is a unique combination of **triangles** which form **hexagons** and occasionally **pentagons**.
  The hexagons and pentagons then form a sphere.
- Adenovirus genes encode proteins which interfere with the expression of host MHC, therefore APCs can not present the virus and the virus evades host immunity.
- Adenovirus causes tumors in animals; and may cause latent infections in humans.

Genus: Adenovirus

Species: Adenovirus serotypes: (47+ types)

- Disease:
  - **1, 2, 3, 5: Intussusception:** in children.
  - **3, 7: Pharyngoconjunctival Fever:**
    Common cause of conjunctivitis and pharyngitis in children.
  - **3, 4, 7: Respiratory Infections; Atypical Pneumonia:**
    In young adults, especially military.
  - **8, 19, 37: Epidemic Keratoconjunctivitis:** in adults.
  - **11, 21: Hemorrhagic Cystitis:** mostly in children.
  - **40, 41: Diarrhea:**
    Common cause of diarrhea in infants.
- Transmission:
  - **Fecal-oral** route.
  - **Respiratory** route.
- Geographic Range: **World-wide**.
- Diagnosis:
  - Based on clinical presentation.
  - Virus isolation, serology, tissue culture, etc. are rarely performed.
- Treatment: symptomatic relief; disease is often self-limited.
- Immunity: post-infectious, long-lasting, type-specific immunity (IgG).
- Vaccine:
  - **Live virus** vaccine is made with **non-attenuated strains 4 and 7**.
    Vaccine comes as an enteric-coated capsule (to withstand stomach acid). After ingestion, the **strains 4 and 7** generated an immune response which builds type-specific antibody. No infection arises because **strains 4 and 7** can only infect the respiratory tract, not the GI tract, due to temperature tropism. Vaccine is used for **military** personnel.

Family: PAPOVA VIRUS

GENERA AND SPECIES:
Human Papillomavirus:
More than 50 serotypes.
Human Polyomavirus:
JC virus
BK virus

GENOME:
DS Circular DNA

SEGMENTATION:
No other segments

NUCLEOCAPSID:
Icosahedral

LOCATION OF REPLICATION:
Nucleus

ENVELOPE:
No Envelope

EFFECT ON HOST CELL:
Variable, depends on strain.

SPECIAL FACTS:
- **Hallmark** of **Human Papillomavirus** infection is **PROLIFERATION.**
- **NOTE:** HPV-1, HPV-2, HPV-6, HPV-11 : have their DNA inserted into the host cells as **episomes.**
- **NOTE:** HPV-16, HPV-18 : have their DNA inserted into the host cells as **integrated into the host DNA.**

Genus: Human Papillomavirus

Species: HPV-1, HPV-2
- Disease: **Common Warts:** Occur on hands, feet. Regress spontaneously.
- Transmission: direct contact.
- Geographic Range: **World-wide.**
- Diagnosis: clinical presentation.
- Treatment: ▪**Salicylic acid-Lactic acid** topical ointment.
  ▪**Cryotherapy.**

Species: HPV-6, HPV-11
- Disease:
  ▪**Anal, Oral, or Genital Warts: "Condyloma Acuminata"**
  Flesh-colored, pedunculated papules which may "accumulate."
  Occur on penis, vagina, cervix, urethra, anus.
  Rarely regress, and often **recur** even after treatment.
  May grow very large during pregnancy or immunosuppression.
  ▪**Malignant transformation:** may occur at sites of infection.
- Transmission:
  ▪**Horizontal** via **sexual contact:** becoming very common.
  ▪**Vertical** during birth via passage through vagina.
- Geographic Range: **World-wide.**
- Diagnosis:
  ▪Clinical presentation.
  ▪**5% Acetic acid:** causes whitening (but not specific for HPV).
- Treatment:
  ▪**Emotional support:** due to relentless nature of infection.
  ▪**Podophyllin; Cryotherapy;** or **Surgery:** for cosmetics.
- Vaccine: none.

Species: HPV-16, HPV-18
- Disease: **Cervical Carcinoma:** can be **fatal.**
- Transmission: horizontal via **sexual contact.**
- Geographic Range: **World-wide.**
- Diagnosis: **Pap smear** shows **Koilocytes.**
- Treatment: surgery.
- Vaccine: none.

Genus: Polyomavirus

Species: JC Virus
- Disease: **PML:**
  Progressive Multifocal Leukoencephalopathy:
  Infection of **oligodendrocytes** leads to progressive demyelination. Occurs mostly in **AIDS** and otherwise **immunocompromised** patients.
  Symptoms: **hemiparesis,** visual field problems, and focal deficits progress to **dementia** and coma.
  PML is **rapidly fatal** (mos.).
- Transmission: most all humans are seropositive.
  Virus remains **latent** in the host **kidney.**
- Geographic Range: **World-wide.**
- Diagnosis:
  ▪**CT scan** shows loss of white matter in cerebrum.
  ▪**Brain biopsy** shows oligodendrocyte basophilic intranuclear inclusion body.
  ▪PCR of **urine** to detect JC Virus DNA.
- Treatment: no effective treatment..
- Vaccine: none.

Species: BK Virus
- Disease: mostly **asymptomatic.**
- Transmission: most all humans are seropositive.
  Virus remains **latent** in the host **kidney.**
- Geographic Range: **World-wide.**
- Diagnosis: PCR of **urine** to detect BK Virus DNA.
- Treatment: none.
- Vaccine: none.

Family: HEPADNAVIRUS

GENERA AND SPECIES:
Hepatitis B Virus:
Hepatitis B
Defective Virus:
Hepatitis D Virus

GENOME:
Partial DS Circular DNA

SEGMENTATION:
No other segments

NUCLEOCAPSID:
Icosahedral

LOCATION OF REPLICATION:
Nucleus

ENVELOPE:
Envelope

EFFECT ON HOST CELL:
Buds from plasma membrane.
No host cell lysis.

SPECIAL FACTS:
- HBV has very unique DNA: it is circular and mostly double stranded, but one section is single stranded (the "missing portion" of DNA).
- HBV has three different forms when found in human blood: whole virions, spherical pieces and filamentous pieces.
- HBV has three different major antigens: **HBsAg** is a protein found on the envelope surface; **HBcAg** and **HBeAg** are proteins found in the capsid core.

PATHOGENESIS: HBV Life Cycle:
1. **HBV** travel in the blood then adhere to host hepatocytes.
2. After entry and uncoating, the viral DNA polymerase replicates the "missing portion" of viral genome double-stranded DNA.
3. Some portions of viral DNA gets integrated into the host genome, other portions serve as templates for mRNA transcription.
4. Some of the newly transcribed mRNA gets "reverse transcribed" into viral genomic DNA by a process similar to Retroviral reverse transcriptase.
5. The virion is formed in the cytoplasm then buds from the hepatocyte plasma membrane.

Genus: Hepatitis B Virus

Species: Hepatitis B (many types)

NOTE: HBV is known as the "**Dane particle**."
- **Disease:**
  - **Asymptomatic:** newly infected people or chronic carriers may remain asymptomatic or **anicteric** (no jaundice).
  - **Acute hepatitis:** after a **2 month incubation period**, symptoms of hepatic inflammation begin such as fever, nausea, right upper quadrant pain, icterus (jaundice), dark urine. Symptoms resolve after 2-3 months. Relapses rarely occur, but the infection may progress to chronic carrier state or chronic active hepatitis
  - **Chronic carrier:** sub-clinical persistence of HBV in host hepatocytes is detected by persistence of HBsAg in blood. Neonatal HBV infections often lead to the chronic carrier state.
  - **Chronic active hepatitis:** prolonged, symptomatic, icteric, persistent infection with HBV usually results from an initially mild infection. Can lead to **liver cirrhosis**. Can be **fatal**.
  - **Fulminant hepatitis:** characterized by rapid progression to liver necrosis. It is acute, severe, symptomatic, and **rapidly fatal**.
  - **Hepatocellular Carcinoma:** may arise in chronic carriers, or in chronic active hepatitis patients. This is **fatal**.
- **Transmission:**
  - **Horizontal** via **sexual contact** and **close personal contact**.
  - **Horizontal** via **IV drug abuse**, sharing needles.
  - **Horizontal** from patient to **health care worker** via needle stick.
  - **Iatrogenic** via **Blood transfusions**, organ transplants, etc.
  - **Vertical mother to child** via **breast milk** or **during birth**.
- **Geographic Range: World-wide.**
- **Diagnosis: serology:**
  - **HBeAg:** indicates active infection, and **transmissibility**.
  - **HBsAg:** indicates active infection; most commonly used test. Continued presence indicates **carrier state**.
  - **HBcAg-specific antibody:** present during **"window period"** after HBsAg disappears and before **HBsAg-specific antibody** appears.
  - Elevated Liver Function Test (LFT); especially ↑**ALT** enzyme.

- **Treatment:**
- **Acute Hepatitis:** symptom relief. **Note:** disappearance of HBeAg and appearance of **HBeAg-specific antibody** indicates end of transmissibility. Disappearance of HBsAg and presence of **HBsAg-specific antibody** indicates end of infection.
- **Chronic Carriers:** education to prevent transmission.
- **Chronic Hepatitis: Interferon-α** is temporarily effective.
- **Chronic Hepatitis** may require liver transplant surgery; but HBV may infect the new liver, due to latency of the virus elsewhere in the host's body.
- **Fulminant Hepatitis** may require liver transplant surgery. The new liver is unlikely to become infected because the HBV is usually restricted to the old liver.
- **Immunity:** post-infectious immunity is long lasting.
- **Vaccine:**
- **Active immunization:** Inactivated HBV particles: spheres and filaments which contain HBsAg.
- **Passive immunization: HBsAg-specific IgG antibody.**
- **Prevention:** abstinence from risky sexual behavior; condoms. Health care workers must use universal precautions.

SEE GRAPHS IN VIRUS CROSS REFERENCE CHAPTER

Family: HEPADNAVIRUS (cont'd)

Please see previous page for HBV presentation.

Even though HDV is an RNA virus, it is included here because it requires components of HBV in order to survive within a human host.

Genus: Hepatitis D Virus

Species: Hepatitis D

NOTE: HDV is known as **"Delta agent"**
(Do not confuse this with HBV known as the "Dane particle")

- Virion:

GENOME: ss(-) Circular RNA
The RNA codes for one protein: HDV antigen (Delta antigen).
HDV is similar to a virioid but can not be considered a viriod.
ENVELOPE: Double Envelope:
Inner layer is HDVAg envelope
Outer layer is HBsAg envelope donated to HDV by HBV.

- Pathogenesis:

HDV is a **"defective" virus** because, in order to be infectious, it requires either **coinfection** concurrently with a new primary HBV infection or **superinfection** upon a **pre-existing chronic or carrier-state** HBV infection. In either case, HBV donates an outer envelope coat to HDV to make HDV a whole, infectious virus.

- Disease:
  - **Chronic carrier state** or Chronic Hepatitis leading to **cirrhosis**.
  - **Fulminant Hepatitis** with **high mortality**.
- Transmission:
  - Restricted to **IV drug abusers** who share needles.
- Geographic Range: **World-wide.**
- Diagnosis: **serology:**
  - **HDV-specific IgM antibody;** or HDV **RNA**.
  - **Coinfection:** HDV-specific IgM and HBcAg-specific IgM are present together in the same serum sample.
  - **Superinfection:** HDV-specific IgM and HBsAg are present together in the same serum sample.
  - Elevated Liver Function Test (LFT): especially ↑**ALT** enzyme.
- Treatment: high dose **Interferon-α** may be helpful.
- Vaccine: no vaccine, no passive immunity.

Family: HERPES VIRUS

GENERA AND SPECIES:

Alpha Virus:
Herpes Simplex Virus 1 (HSV-1)
Herpes Simplex Virus 2 (HSV-2)
Varacella Zoster Virus (VZV)
Beta Virus:
Cytomegalovirus (CMV)
Gamma Virus:
Epstein-Barr Virus (EBV)
Human Herpes Virus-6 (HHV-6)

GENOME:
DS linear DNA

SEGMENTATION:
No other segments

NUCLEOCAPSID:
Icosahedral

LOCATION OF REPLICATION:
Nucleus

ENVELOPE:
Envelope

EFFECT ON HOST CELL:
The only **VIRUS** which buds from the host cell **NUCLEUS**.
Escape from host cell is through a **pore** or else causes **host cell lysis**.

SPECIAL FACTS:
▪All Herpes viruses can cause persistent and **latent** infections:
initial infection is known as the **primary** infection; recrudescent or relapsing infection is known as the **secondary** infection.
▪All Herpes viruses tend to form **intra-nuclear inclusions**.
▪Size comparison of Herpes virus **genomes**:
From **smallest to largest**: VZV HSV HHV6 EBV CMV
▪Herpes viruses spread from infected cell to neighboring cell; they do not survive long extracellularly.

Genus: Alpha Virus

Species: HSV-1, HSV-2: (Herpes Simplex Virus 1,2)

●HSV-1:
▪**Gingivostomatitis, Herpes Labialis** (cold sores):
Painful, itchy, relapsing vesicular lesions of lips/mouth.
▪**Keratoconjunctivitis**
▪**Herpetic Whitlow**: vesicular skin lesions on finger.
▪Adult **Necrotizing Encephalitis**: rapidly **fatal**.
●HSV-2:
▪**Herpes Genitalis**: painful, itchy, relapsing vesicular lesions of genitalia, groin, anus.
▪**Herpetic Whitlow**: vesicular skin lesions on finger.
▪**Neonatal skin lesions and Encephalitis**: rapidly fatal.
▪**Aseptic meningitis**.
●Transmission: (primary incubation: 2-10 days).
Note: infectious virus may be shed even when vesicles are absent.
▪**HSV-1: Horizontal** via **direct contact**.
▪**HSV-2: Horizontal** via **sexual contact**.
▪**HSV-2: Vertical** from mother to newborn **during birth**.
▪Health care workers are at risk for both HSV-1, HSV-2.
●Diagnosis:
▪**Tzanck smear**: shows **multinucleated giant cells**.
Method: scrape skin at base of vesicle, mount on slide, fix in methyl alcohol, stain with Giemsa or Wright stain.
▪**Brain biopsy** may be needed for **encephalitis** diagnosis.
▪**CSF** may show **blood** in HSV **meningitis** cases.
●Treatment: **Acyclovir**: activated by **viral thymidine kinase**;
serves to block **viral DNA polymerase**; helps symptoms. **No cure**.
Emotional support is necessary due to relentless nature of infection.
Education is necessary to prevent spread, and to protect neonate.
●Immunity: infections may become **persistent** or **latent**.
▪**HSV-1** tends to be latent in **Trigeminal sensory ganglia**.
▪**HSV-2** tends to be latent in **Lumbo-Sacral sensory ganglia**.
●Prevention: No vaccine. **C-section** at birth may protect neonates.
Condoms may **not** be effective to stop transmission.

Species: VZV: (Varicella Zoster Virus)

●**Chicken Pox**: (late winter season)
▪**Itchy, centripetal, vesicular rash** appears on trunk first, then spreads. Rash described as **"dew drop on rose petal."**
Rash stages: papule, vesicle, crust. Note: lesions at different stages may be present at the same time. Benign, self-limited.
▪**Cellulitis** superinfection by *S. pyogenese*, or *S. aureus*.
▪**Pneumonitis** in **immunocompromised**, can be **fatal**.
▪**Hemorrhagic chicken pox** in childhood **leukemia**.
▪**Reye Syndrome** may arise in children who use **aspirin**.
●**Herpes zoster**: "Shingles"
▪Reactivation of latent VZV from sensory ganglia occurs due to stress, immunocomromised state, old age.
▪Painful vesicular skin lesions arise within **dermatomes**.
▪**Post-Herpetic Neuralgia** is a condition of intermittent nerve pain that can last for years after the zoster rash heals.
●Transmission: (primary incubation: 1-2 weeks): **mostly children**.
▪**Horizontal** via **respiratory route**: **highly contagious**. Patients are infectious at 48 hrs prior to rash, continuing until all vesicles crusted.
▪Contact with Herpes zoster patient can cause chicken pox.
●Diagnosis: **Tzanck smear**: shows **multinucleated giant cells**.
●Treatment: **isolation** required of patient and seronegative contacts.
Skin must be kept **clean** to prevent superinfection. **Topical lotion** or oral antihistamines may help for pruritus. **Acyclovir** may be helpful, especially in **immunocompromised**. Must **not use aspirin**.
Tricyclic antidepressants are used for post-herpetic neuralgia pain.
●Immunity: post-infectious immunity is long lasting, however initial chicken pox infection becomes **latent**: relapses as **zoster**.
▪VZV tends to be latent in **Trigeminal sensory ganglia**, sometimes cervical-thoracic dorsal-root sensory ganglia. (Rarely ventral horn.)
●Vaccine: ▪**Active immunization:** Oka-strain **live** VZV.
Must not be used in immunocompromised or pregnant patients.
▪**Passive immunization: VZV-specific IgG antibody** (VZIG, VIP).
Use within 96 hrs of exposure; for immunocompromised or pregnant.

Family: HERPES VIRUS (cont'd)

Genus: Beta Virus

Species: CMV: (Cytomegalovirus) (only one serotype)
- Diseases:
  - **Most** CMV infections are **asymptomatic.**
  - **CMV Infectious Mononucleosis: "Heterophile-NEG"**
  Symptoms: lymphocytosis with atypical lymphocytes, fever, and hepatosplenomegaly; 20-30 yr old age group.
  - **CMV Retinitis/ Blindness** in **immunocompromised** patients; common in **AIDS** patients with **CD4 count<50.** Funduscopic exam: "pizza pie retina."
  - **Interstitial pneumonitis** in immunocompromised.
  - **CMV Hepatitis** in immunocompromised.
  - **Cytomegalic Inclusion Disease** (Congenital CMV): **Encephalitis** with brain calcifications; may give rise to seizures, mental retardation, and nerve **deafness.**
- Transmission: (primary incubation: 1-2 months).

Note: most humans are infected with CMV.
  - **Horizontal** via **sexual** or **intimate contact**: (present in semen, cervical fluids, saliva, urine, etc).
  - **Iatrogenic** from organ transplant or blood products.
  - **Vertical** from mother to fetus **transplacentally in utero** causes **congenital infection.** Mild, vertically transmitted, infection may occur in the neonate during delivery due to vaginal secretions, or post-partum due to breast feeding.
  - **Reactivation** of latent CMV (**"secondary CMV"**) often occurs as consequence of immunocompromised state.
- Diagnosis:
  - **Serology: CMV-specific IgM or IgG**
  - **Tissue samples: "Owl-Eye" nuclear/cytoplasmic inclusion.**
  - **CT scan:** shows focal **calcifications in brain.**
- Treatment: there is no effective treatment of CMV infection. Either **Ganciclovir** or **Foscarnet** is used for **CMV retinitis** and for **transplant** patients, but **relapse** occurs when treatment is halted.
- Immunity: infections may become **persistent** or **latent.**
  - **CMV** tends to be latent in **many organs** and in some **leukocytes.**
- Vaccine: none.

Genus: Gamma Virus

Species: EBV: (Epstein-Barr Virus)
- Diseases:
  - **Asymptomatic** in children.
  - **EBV Infectious Mononucleosis: "Heterophile-POS"**
  Symptoms: lymphocytosis with atypical lymphocytes, fever, hepatitis, **splenomegaly**, pharyngitis with **exudate**, coated tongue, anorexia, swollen tonsils, and **fatigue.** Occurs mostly in the 15-20 yr old "**college**" age group. Infection is usually benign and self-limited.
  - **Cancer associations:**
    - **Burkett's Lymphoma** in Africa.
    - **Nasopharyngeal Carcinoma** in China.

Note: EBV replicates primarily within B-cells; therefore T-cells proliferate as the host response.
- Transmission: (primary incubation: 1-2 months).
  - **Horizontal** via **oral route: intimate contact**; **kissing** (saliva).
- Diagnosis:
  - **Serology: EBV capsid-antigen-specific IgM antibody.**
  - **Serology: Heterophile-agglutinin** (Monospot test): **POS.**
  - **Peripheral Smear:** shows **atypical T-lymphocytes**: The T-lymphocytes attack B-lymphocytes.
  - **Elevated Liver Function Test** (LFT): especially ↑**ALT**
- Treatment:
  - **Aspirin** or Acetaminophen for constitutional symptoms.
  - **Avoid sports** or excessive activity: may **rupture spleen.**

Note: Avoid ampicillin: it causes non-itchy maculopapular rash.
- Immunity: infections may become **persistent** or **latent.**
  - **EMV** tends to be latent in **B-lymphocytes.**
- Vaccine: none.

Species: HHV-6 (Human Herpesvirus 6)
- **Roseola** (exanthem subitum): Mostly **children** 6mos-12mos.
- Symptoms: sudden onset of **high fever** which lasts 3 days. Pink, rose-color **rash** begins on **trunk** when fever ends.
- Horizontal transmission via **respiratory route.**
- Treatment: symptomatic relief; infection is brief and self-limited.

Family: POX VIRUS

GENERA AND SPECIES:
Orthopoxvirus:
Vaccinia virus
Variola virus
Unclassified:
Molluscum contagiosum virus

GENOME:
DS linear DNA

SEGMENTATION:
No other segments

NUCLEOCAPSID:
Complicated

LOCATION OF REPLICATION:
The only **DNA virus** to replicate in the **CYTOPLASM**.

ENVELOPE:
Double Envelope

EFFECT ON HOST CELL:
Poxvirus causes **no host cell lysis** and **does not bud** from host cell.

SPECIAL FACTS:
- Since **Poxviruses** are the only DNA viruses that do not replicate in the host cell nucleus, they must carry their own DNA-dependent-RNA-polymerase enzymes.
- **Poxviruses** cause **no host cell lysis** and **do not bud** from host plasma membrane. The unique double-layered envelope is acquired at the host **golgi** apparatus.
- **Poxviruses** are the largest and most complex viruses.

Genus: Orthopoxvirus

Species: Vaccinia
- Disease: **Cowpox:** self-limited infection manifest by vesicular lesion on fingers due to milking of infected cows by hand.
  - Live attenuated virus vaccine made with **Vaccinia** virus is used to protect against smallpox. This vaccine has some **rare side-effects:** Vesicular rash; encephalitis; viremia in immunocompromised, Vaccinia Necrosum (necrosis and gangrene at inoculation site progresses throughout the body; this can be fatal).
- Treatment: Vaccinia immunoglobulin is sometimes effective.

Species: Variola (Smallpox Virus: two strains)
- **Pathogenesis:**
  1. **Variola** virus first establishes infection in respiratory tract.
  2. It spreads to blood as primary viremia.
  3. It infects internal organs.
  4. It infects the skin as a vesicular rash.
- Disease: **Smallpox:**
  The **vesicular rash** begins on face and trunk then spreads rapidly to extremities. The rash **stages:** macules, papules, vesicles, then crust. This rash is differentiated from the rash of chicken pox because: in smallpox, all lesions are at the **same stage of development**; but in chicken pox, lesions of various stages will be present concurrently.
- **Strains: Variola Major:** 50% mortality. **Variola minor:** 1% mortality.
- Transmission: horizontal via **respiratory** route.
- Geographic Range: **none.**
- NOTE: **Smallpox has been eliminated due to effective prevention.**
- Diagnosis: characteristic clinical presentation. Virus isolation.
- Treatment: symptomatic relief; sometimes **Variola** immunoglobulin.
- Immunity: post-infectious, long-lasting immunity (IgG).
- Vaccine: **Live, attenuated Vaccinia virus:** (now only for military use).
- NOTE: the successful elimination of smallpox (last case 1977) is due to:
  1. Humans are the only reservoir
  2. Safe vaccine causes rapid antibody production.
  3. There are only two serotypes (sometimes considered one type).
  4. Clinically easy to recognize (no carrier or sub-clinical states).

Genus: Unclassified Poxvirus

Species: Molluscum contagiosum virus
- Disease:
  - **Genital Tumors:** benign, self-limited, pedunculated, firm, pink papules arise in genital areas of adults.
  - **Disseminated:** infection in **immunocompromised** progresses from genital tumors to systemic infection. Large skin tumors may arise anywhere.
  - **Skin tumors:** small, benign, self-limited, wart-like cutaneous papules may occur in children and adults.
- Transmission:
  - Horizontal via direct contact.
  - Horizontal via **sexual** contact.
- Geographic Range: **World-wide.**
- Diagnosis: electron microscopy of biopsy.
- Treatment:
  - **Local lesions:** surgery, laser, cryotherapy.
  - **Disseminated:** no treatment.
- Vaccine: none.

Chapter 17

RNA VIRUSES

Positive-sense
Single-strand linear RNA
Icosahedral
No envelope
Picornavirus
Rhinovirus Coryza (common cold)
Enterovirus
    Coxsackie A Aseptic meningitis
        Hand-foot-mouth disease
    Coxsackie B Aseptic meningitis
        Pleurodynia
        Myopericarditis
    Echo Aseptic meningitis
    Enterovirus 70 Conjunctivitis
    Enterovirus 71 Encephalitis
    Hepatitis A Acute Hepatitis
    Polio Aseptic meningitis
        Polio
Calicivirus
    Norwalk virus Gastroenteritis
    Hepatitis E Acute Hepatitis

Double-strand linear RNA
Segmented
Icosahedral
No envelope
Reovirus
    Rotavirus Diarrhea
    Coltivirus Colorado tick fever

Positive-sense
Single-strand linear RNA
Icosahedral
Envelope
Togavirus
    Alphavirus
        Eastern equine encephalitis
        Western equine encephalitis
        Venezuelan equine encephalitis
    Rubivirus
        Rubella German measles
            Congenital Rubella
Flavivirus
    Mosquito-borne epidemic types
        Yellow fever virus
        Dengue fever virus
        St. Louis encephalitis virus
        Japanese encephalitis virus
    Hepatitis C Acute Hepatitis
           Chronic Hepatitis
           Carrier State Hepatitis
           Hepatocellular carcinoma

Positive-sense
Single-strand linear RNA
Helical
Envelope
Coronavirus Coryza (common cold)

Negative-sense
Single-strand linear RNA
Helical
Envelope
Rhabdovirus
    Lyssavirus
        Rabies Rabies
Paramyxovirus
    Paramyxo
        Mumps Mumps
        Parainfluenza Croup
    Morbillivirus
        Measles Measles
    Pneumovirus
        RSV Bronchiolitis
Filovirus
    Ebola virus Hemorrhagic fever
    Marbug virus Hemorrhagic fever

Negative-sense
Single-strand linear RNA
Segmented
Helical
Envelope
Orthomyxovirus
    Influenza A Flu, Atypical pneumonia
        Reye syndrome
    Influenza B Flu, Reye syndrome
    Influenza C URI

Negative-sense
Single-stranded circular RNA
Segmented
Helical
Envelope
Arenavirus
    Lymphocytic Choriomeningitis
        Aseptic meningitis
    Lassa Fever virus
Bunyavirus
    California encephalitis virus
    LaCrosse virus

Positive-sense-non-infectious
DIPLOID segmented
Single-strand linear RNA
Complex nucleocapsid
Envelope
Retrovirus
Oncovirus
    HTLV-1 T-cell Leukemia/Lymphoma
        Tropical spastic paraparesis
    HTLV-2 Hairy cell Leukemia
Lentivirus
    HIV-1 ARC, AIDS, malignancies
        Opportunistic infections
    HIV-2 AIDS-like infection
Spumavirus
    Human foamy virus Asymptomatic

Family: PICORNAVIRUS

GENERA AND SPECIES:
Rhinovirus:
  100 types
Enterovirus:
  Coxsackie A virus
  Coxsackie B virus
  Echo virus
  Enteroviruses
  Hepatitis A virus
  Polio virus

GENOME:
ss+ linear RNA
Infectious RNA

SEGMENTATION:
No other segments

NUCLEOCAPSID:
Icosahedral

LOCATION OF REPLICATION:
Cytoplasm

ENVELOPE:
No Envelope

EFFECT ON HOST CELL:
Causes **host cell lysis**

PATHOGENESIS:
Horizontal transmission (except Rhinovirus) is fecal-oral. In general, the GI tract becomes colonized, the Peyers patches get infiltrated, then viremia carries the virus to sites of focal involvement. Usually summer/autumn.

Genus: Rhinovirus

Species: 1-100 (100 types)
- **Disease:**
  - **Common Cold: Coryza**
    Rhinoviruses grow best at 33°C so infection is limited to the upper airway.
- **Transmission:** respiratory route; during winter.
- **Diagnosis:** clinical presentation.
- **Treatment:** symptom relief; disease is self-limited.
- **Immunity:** post-infectious, type-specific immunity (IgG).
- **Vaccine:** none.

Genus: Enterovirus

Species: Coxsackie A (many types)
- **Disease:** (mucus membrane and skin manifestations)
  - **Aseptic Meningitis.**
  - **Hand-foot-mouth Disease:** vesicular rash on hands, feet, with ulcerations in mouth.
  - **Herpangina:** vesicular eruption in throat.
- **Transmission:** **fecal-oral**, viremia. Mostly in **children**.
- **Diagnosis:** clinical presentation, sometimes cell culture.
- **Treatment:** symptom relief; disease is often self-limited.
- **Immunity:** post-infectious, type-specific immunity (IgG).
- **Vaccine:** none.

Species: Coxsackie B (many types)
- **Disease:** (organ dysfunction)
  - **Aseptic Meningitis:** common.
  - **Pleurodynia** ("devil's grip"): pleuritic chest pain.
  - **Myopericarditis:** can be **rapidly fatal**.
  - **Pancreatic damage** may lead to diabetes.
- **Transmission:** **fecal-oral**, viremia. Mostly in **children**.
- **Diagnosis:** clinical presentation, cell culture.
- **Treatment:** symptom relief; disease is often self-limited.
- **Immunity:** post-infectious, type-specific immunity (IgG).
- **Vaccine:** none.

Species: Echo (many types)
- **Disease:**
  - **Aseptic Meningitis:** #1 causative organism.
  - **Neonatal Encephalitis** and **Sepsis:** can be **fatal**.
  - **Neonatal Fulminant Hepatitis:** mostly **fatal**.
  - **Diarrhea**.
- **Transmission:** **fecal-oral**, viremia. Mostly in **children**.
- **Diagnosis:** clinical presentation, cell culture.
- **Treatment:** symptom relief; disease is often self-limited.
- **Immunity:** post-infectious, type-specific immunity (IgG).
- **Vaccine:** none.

Species: Enterovirus 70
- **Disease: Acute Hemorrhagic Conjunctivitis:** common, highly contagious, transient. Sometimes also caused by Coxsackie A24

Species: Enterovirus 71
- **Disease: Paralysis** and **Encephalitis:** can be **fatal**.

Species: Hepatitis A = Enterovirus 72 (one type)
- **Disease: Acute Hepatitis:** hepatic inflammation is mostly asymptomatic in children but causes fever, elevated Liver Function Test, jaundice, dark urine in adults. **No chronic sequelae**, and **no carrier state**.
- **Transmission:** **fecal-oral**; mostly **children**; world-wide, **USA**
- **Diagnosis:** ↑**ALT** (LFT), **Hepatitis A-specific IgM**.
- **Treatment:** symptom relief; disease is self-limited.
- **Immunity:** post-infectious, long-lasting immunity (IgG).
- **Vaccine: Active immunity** with **inactivated virus** vaccine. **Passive immunity** with IgG immunoglobulin.

Species: Polio (three types)
- **Disease:** (polio infection is very **rare**)
  - **Aseptic Meningitis:** common, non-paralytic.
  - **Polio Myelitis:** necrosis of **anterior horn cells** leads to **paralysis**; may extend to bulbar respiratory areas. Can be **fatal**.
- **Transmission:** **fecal-oral**, viremia. Occurs mostly in **children**.
- **Diagnosis:** clinical presentation, isolate virus, serology.
- **Treatment:** symptom relief; respiratory support. Normal function may return over several months.
- **Immunity:** post-infectious, type-specific immunity (IgG).
- **Vaccine:** both vaccines are effective to generate Ig M and IgG:
  - **Salk IPV: dead virus**. No IgA is created. The GI tract is then vulnerable to infection but infection can not progress.
  - **Sabin OPV: live virus**. IgA is created to protect the GI tract. Vaccine may cause disease in immunocompromised: if given to compromised patient or to children in the household who may shed the virus after vaccination.

Family: CALICIVIRUS

GENERA AND SPECIES:
Gastroenteritis group:
    Norwalk Virus
Hepatitis Group:
    Hepatitis E Virus

GENOME:
ss+ linear RNA
Infectious RNA

SEGMENTATION:
No other segments

NUCLEOCAPSID:
Icosahedral

LOCATION OF REPLICATION:
Cytoplasm

ENVELOPE:
No Envelope

EFFECT ON HOST CELL:
Causes **host cell lysis**

Gastroenteritis Group:

Species: Norwalk Virus
- Disease:
  - **Gastroenteritis:** nausea, abdominal cramps, vomiting, diarrhea lasting for 3 days. Infection by Norwalk is very common, can cause epidemics.
- Transmission:
  - **Fecal-oral.**
  - Some people are not susceptible (do not absorb it).
- Geographic Range: **World-wide.**
- Diagnosis:
  - Immune electron microscopy of stool sample.
  - Serology: **Norwalk-specific IgM antibody.**
  - Culture has not been achieved.
- Treatment: oral fluid replacement.
- Immunity: post-infectious immunity is **not long lasting**. **Re-infection** is possible after several months.
- Vaccine: none.

Hepatitis Group:

Species: Hepatitis E (one type)
- Disease:
  - **Acute Hepatitis:** hepatic inflammation is mostly asymptomatic in children, but causes fever, elevated Liver Function Test, jaundice, dark urine in adults. **No chronic sequelae**, and **no carrier state.**
  - **Fulminant Hepatitis of Pregnant Women: Fatal** for mother if infected in **first trimester.**
- Transmission:
  - **Fecal-oral**; mostly **adults.**
  - SE Asia, India, Africa, Mexico.
- Diagnosis:
  - **↑ALT**; process of elimination of other causes.
  - Immune electron microscopy of stool sample;
  - **Hepatitis E-specific IgM** test not widely available.
- Treatment: symptom relief; disease is self-limited.
- Immunity:
  - Post-infectious immunity may **not** be long lasting.
- Vaccine: Passive immunity with IgG immunoglobulin.

Family: REOVIRUS

GENERA AND SPECIES:
Rotavirus: (11 segments RNA)
   Rotavirus A, B, C
Coltivirus: (12 segments RNA)
   Colorado tick fever

GENOME:
DS linear RNA

SEGMENTATION:
10-12 RNA segments

NUCLEOCAPSID:
Icosahedral
Double-layer

LOCATION OF REPLICATION:
Cytoplasm

ENVELOPE:
No Envelope

EFFECT ON HOST CELL:
Causes **host cell lysis**

SPECIAL FACTS:

- **Double-layer capsid:** electron microscopy shows as **"wheel"** structure.
- Original virus remains intact within host cells: **no eclipse period,**
     because the virus does not go through the uncoating process.
- Many RNA segments allow for **resortment** of genetic material; this may
     lead to antigenic variation.

Genus: Rotavirus

Species: Rotavirus Groups A, B, C

- Disease:
  - **Gastroenteritis:**
  Rotavirus is the #1 cause of Diarrhea in children.
  Diarrhea is a significant cause of **fatality** in children.
- Transmission:
  - **Fecal-oral.**
  - **Winter** season.
- Geographic Range: **World-wide.**
- Diagnosis:
  - Detection of Rotavirus in stool sample by **ELISA.**
  - Immune electron microscopy of stool sample.
- Treatment: oral fluid and electrolyte replacement with specially balanced formulas.
- Immunity: post-infectious immunity is **not long lasting.**
  Re-infection is possible after several months, most likely due to antigenic variation from resortment.
- Vaccine: none.

Genus: Coltivirus

Species: Colorado Tick Fever (many types)
(Formerly classified in the genus Orbivirus)

- Disease:
  - **Colorado Tick Fever:** biphasic symptoms:
  high fever, rash, nausea, vomiting; then remission for a few days; **fever** then returns but symptoms usually resolve in a few weeks. The unique aspect of viremia with Colorado Tick Fever is that the virus survives **within red blood cells.**
- Transmission: **Vector** = tick
             Reservoir = squirrels, chipmunks
             Hosts = Humans
  - Late **spring**, early summer.
- Geographic Range: **Western North America.**
- Diagnosis:
  - Direct immunofluorescent stain of virus in RBCs.
  - Serology.
- Treatment: supportive care; acetaminophen for fever.
- Immunity: post-infectious, type-specific immunity (IgG).
- Vaccine: none.

Family: TOGAVIRUS

GENERA AND SPECIES:

Alphavirus:
Eastern equine encephalitis
Western equine encephalitis
Venezuelan equine encephalitis

Rubivirus:
Rubella virus

GENOME:
ss+ linear RNA
Infectious RNA

SEGMENTATION:
No other segments

NUCLEOCAPSID:
Icosahedral
C -protein only

LOCATION OF REPLICATION:
Cytoplasm

ENVELOPE:
Envelope
H-protein spike

EFFECT ON HOST CELL:
Buds from plasma membrane.
No host cell lysis.

Genus: Alphavirus

Species: Eastern equine encephalitis
- Disease: **Encephalitis:** CNS infection with high fever; 50% **fatal**. Can cause **epidemics**.
- Transmission: **Vector** = mosquito
  Reservoir = birds
  Hosts = Humans, horses
- Geographic Range: **south-east USA**, very rare.
- Diagnosis: virus isolation, serology.
- Treatment: intensive supportive care.
- Immunity: post-infectious, type-specific immunity (IgG).
- Vaccine: for animals only.

Species: Western equine encephalitis
- Disease: **Encephalitis:** CNS infection with high fever; can be **fatal**. Can cause **epidemics**.
- Transmission: **Vector** = mosquito
  Reservoir = birds
  Hosts = Humans, horses
- Geographic Range: **western USA**, rare.
- Diagnosis: virus isolation, serology.
- Treatment: intensive supportive care.
- Immunity: post-infectious, type-specific immunity (IgG).
- Vaccine: for animals only.

Species: Venezuela equine encephalitis
- Disease: **Encephalitis:** CNS infection with high fever; can be **fatal**. Can cause **epidemics**.
- Transmission: **Vector** = mosquito
  Reservoir = birds
  Hosts = Humans, horses
- Geographic Range: **South** and **Central America**, common.
- Diagnosis: virus isolation, serology.
- Treatment: intensive supportive care.
- Immunity: post-infectious, type-specific immunity (IgG).
- Vaccine: for animals only.

Genus: Rubivirus

Species: Rubella virus (only one type)
- Disease:
  - **German Measles: fever** and maculopapular **rash** on **face** may arise simultaneously; then rash spreads to the extremities and lasts for 3 days. Can cause **epidemics**.
  - **Congenital Rubella: Rubella virus** is a **teratogen**, especially when mother is infected in **first trimester**. Viremia crosses placenta to cause disease in the fetus:
    - **Heart:** patent ductus arteriosus (PDA)
    - **Eyes:** cataracts, glaucoma.
    - **CNS:** mental retardation, **deafness**.
- Note: children infected in-utero may continue to **shed** the virus for many months. This poses **risk to pregnant** women and to **immunocomromised** people.
- Transmission:
  German Measles: **respiratory** route, viremia
  Congenital: **transplacental** vertical transmission in-utero.
- Diagnosis: clinical presentation, cell-culture, serology shows **Rubella-specific IgM antibody**.
- Treatment: symptom relief.
- Immunity: post-infectious, type-specific immunity (IgG).
- Vaccine:
  - **Live virus:** as part of **MMR** vaccine.
- Note: Vaccine may cause disease in immunocompromised: if given to compromised patient or to children in the household who may shed the virus after vaccination. However, MMR is given in **HIV** infected patients.

Family: FLAVIVIRUS

GENERA AND SPECIES:	GENOME:
Mosquito-Borne Epidemic Types	**ss+ linear RNA**
Yellow Fever Virus	**Infectious RNA**
Dengue Fever Virus	
St. Louis Encephalitis Virus	SEGMENTATION:
Japanese Encephalitis Virus	No other segments
Hepatitis C Virus:	
Hepatitis C Virus	NUCLEOCAPSID:
	Icosahedral

LOCATION OF REPLICATION:	ENVELOPE:
Cytoplasm	**Envelope**
EFFECT ON HOST CELL:	**E-, M-protein** spikes
Buds from plasma membrane.	
No host cell lysis.	

Mosquito-Borne Epidemic Types:

Species: Yellow Fever Virus (only one type)
- Disease:
    - **Yellow Fever:** begins with **fever** and headache; then remission for a few days; then fever again with **jaundice** and **hemorrhage** (e.g. hematemesis). Symptoms range from mild to severe; can be **fatal**.
- Transmission: **Vector** = mosquito
    - **Reservoir** = monkeys ("jungle fever")
    - **Hosts** = Humans ("urban fever")
- Geographic Range: **South America** and **Africa**.
- Diagnosis: virus isolation, serology.
- Treatment: intensive supportive care; medications such as acetaminophen (fever) and antacid (stomach bleed).
- Immunity: post-infectious, type-specific immunity (IgG).
- Vaccine:
    - **Live virus:** given every 10 years.

Species: Dengue Fever Virus (4 types)
- Disease:
    - **Dengue Fever ("Breakbone Fever"):** biphasic symptoms: **high fever**, rash, nausea, bone pain; then remission for a few days; fever returns with a new maculopapular rash. Symptoms resolve in 2 weeks.
    - **Hemorrhagic Fever:** high fever, hypotension due to hemorrhage (e.g. GI tract bleed, etc.), shock. Severe illness; can be **fatal**.
- Transmission: **Vector** = mosquito
    - **Reservoir** = Humans
- Geographic Range: **World-wide**.
- Diagnosis: virus isolation, serology.
- Treatment: intensive supportive care; fluid replacement.
- Immunity: post-infectious, type-specific immunity (IgG).
- Vaccine: none.

Species: St. Louis Encephalitis Virus
- Disease:
    - **Encephalitis:** CNS infection; symptoms range from asymptomatic to severe illness (especially in the elderly). Can be **fatal**, especially in the elderly.
- Transmission: **Vector** = mosquito
    - **Reservoir** = birds
    - **Hosts** = Humans
- Geographic Range: **North America**.
- Diagnosis: virus isolation, serology.
- Treatment: intensive supportive care; anticonvulsants.
- Immunity: post-infectious, type-specific immunity (IgG).
- Vaccine: none

Species: Japanese Encephalitis Virus
- Disease:
    - **Encephalitis:** CNS infection; symptoms range from asymptomatic to severe illness (especially in children). Can be **fatal**, but mostly asymptomatic.
- Transmission: **Vector** = mosquito
    - **Reservoir** = birds, pigs
    - **Hosts** = Humans
- Geographic Range: **Asia** and **India**
- Diagnosis: virus isolation, serology.
- Treatment: intensive supportive care; anticonvulsants.
- Immunity: post-infectious, type-specific immunity (IgG).
- Vaccine:
    - **Dead virus:** used in south east Asia.

FLAVIVIRUS continues on the next page.

Family: FLAVIVIRUS (Cont'd)

Genus: Hepatitis C Virus

Species: Hepatitis C

NOTE: HCV is known as the "Post-Transfusion Hepatitis."

● Disease:
- **Asymptomatic:** newly infected people or chronic carriers may remain asymptomatic or **anicteric** (no jaundice).
- **Acute hepatitis:** after a **6 week incubation period**, symptoms of hepatic inflammation begin such as fever, nausea, right upper quadrant pain, icterus (jaundice), dark urine. Symptoms resolve after 2-3 months. **Relapses commonly occur**, and infection often progresses to the chronic carrier state or chronic active hepatitis
- **Neonatal** HCV infection is **rare**.
- **Chronic carrier:** sub-clinical persistence of HCV in host hepatocytes is detected by serology.
- **Chronic active hepatitis:** prolonged, symptomatic, icteric, persistent HCV infection usually follows a course of relapses and remissions. Can lead to **liver cirrhosis**. Can be **fatal**.
- **Fulminant hepatitis:** characterized by rapid progression to liver necrosis is **rare** with HCV infection.
- **Hepatocellular Carcinoma:** may arise in chronic carriers, or in chronic active hepatitis patients. This is **fatal**.

● Transmission:
- **Horizontal** via **IV drug abuse**, sharing needles.
- **Iatrogenic** via **Blood transfusions**, organ transplants, etc.
- Horizontal transmission (via sexual contact) and vertical transmission are each possible, but unlikely to occur.

● Geographic Range: **World-wide.**

● Diagnosis: fabricated HCV **antigen** can **indirectly** detect serum antibody, **real** HCV **antigen** is **not** available to measure **real HCV-specific antibody.**
- **ELISA tests for "Recombinant HCV-specific antibody:"**
  - NS4 sequence: "c100-3" antigen.
  - NS3 sequence: "c33-C" or "c200" antigens.
  - Core Protein: "c22-3" antigen.
- **Confirmatory test for "Recombinant HCV-specific antibody:"**
  - **RIBA** (Recombinant immunoblot assay).
- Elevated Liver Function Test (LFT); especially ↑**ALT** enzyme.

● Treatment:
- **Acute Hepatitis:** symptom relief, symptoms are usually mild.
- **Chronic Carriers:** education to prevent transmission.
- **Chronic Hepatitis: Interferon-α** is temporarily effective.
- **Chronic Hepatitis** may require liver transplant surgery, but HCV may infect the new liver, due to latency of the virus elsewhere in the host's body.
- **Fulminant Hepatitis** may require liver transplant surgery. The new liver is unlikely to become infected because the HCV is usually restricted to the old liver.

● Immunity: post-infectious immunity is ineffective.

● Vaccine: none.

SPECIAL FACTS:

- HCV infection is nearly indistinguishable from HBV on a clinical basis. However, HCV is more likely to cause **persistent** and chronic infection.
- Diagnostic tests do not include tests for **HCV-specific antibodies** because the immune system, for unknown reasons, can not launch an effective defense.
- The details about the life cycle of HCV are unknown.
- Much is unknown about HCV.

Family: RHABDOVIRUS

GENERA AND SPECIES:

Lyssavirus:
Rabies virus

GENOME:

ss(-) linear RNA

SEGMENTATION:
No other segments

NUCLEOCAPSID:
Helical

LOCATION OF REPLICATION:
Cytoplasm

ENVELOPE:
**Envelope
BULLET-SHAPE**

EFFECT ON HOST CELL:
Buds from plasma membrane.
No host cell lysis.

SPECIAL FACTS:
- **Negri Bodies:** eosinophilic **cytoplasmic inclusion bodies** in the **neurons** of the **hippocampus** infected by Rabies Virus
- **NOTE:**
Rabies Virus surface protein antigens have the ability to move from the virion surface to the virion interior to **escape host antibody opsonization**.
- **NOTE:**
Rabies Virus infection is the **most deadly** infection known: **untreated mortality is 100%.**

PATHOGENESIS:
- **Zoonotic** transmission occurs via **animal bite**. First, **sensory neurons** are infected. The Rabies Virus moves to the **CNS** by axonal transport. Virus multiplies in the CNS then travels down **cranial nerves** and other **peripheral nerves** to various organs and to **salivary glands**.
- **Horizontal** transmission occurs, especially among **health care workers** by contact with **bodily fluids** (saliva, tears, urine) from infected patient.

Genus: Lyssavirus

Species: Rabies virus (many types)
- Disease: **Rabies:**
  - **Hydrophobia:** painful swallowing, foaming at mouth: due to cranial nerve involvement. **Dehydration** from nausea with vomiting.
  - **Encephalitis:** demyelination and neuron death: confusion and lethargy.
  - **Seizures, coma, death.**
- Transmission: **Zoonotic** via animal bite: **Horizontal** via bodily secretions:
  - Bite from **unprovoked encounter** with an unusually **aggressive** animal.
  - Animals are infectious one week before they die.
  - Bats may remain asymtomatc while infectious.
  - Birds, opossum, rabbits, reptiles, rodents, squirrels, do **not** carry Rabies
  - **Horizontal** via saliva, tears, urine, CSF. **Health care workers** are at risk.
- Geographic Range: **World-wide.**
- Diagnosis:
  - History of **unprovoked** animal bite is sufficient evidence.
  - There are no diagnostic tests prior to onset of symptoms.
  - Once symptoms begin, diagnostic tests are useless because death is certain.
  - **Negri Bodies** seen in brain at **autopsy** of human or animal.
  - **Rabies Virus-specific antigen** immunofluorescence of corneal scrapings, or of skin can be done.
- Treatment:
  - Step #1: **wash** the bite site thoroughly.
  - Step #2: **passive immunization** by **systemic** injection of **HRIG** (Human Rabies immune globulin), one dose (IM in gluteal).
  - Step #3: inject **HRIG** around the **bite site**.
  - Step #4: **active immunization** with **HDCV** or **RVA dead virus vaccine** given (IM in deltoid) on days 0, 3, 7, 14, and 28 following bite.
  - **Note:** injections should begin within 48 hours, but no later than 4-5 days.
- Immunity: antibodies are slow to develop and are ineffective once symptoms begin.
- Vaccine: • Passive immunization **HRIG** (Human Rabies immune globulin)
  - Active immunization **HDCV** or **RVA**: **dead virus** vaccines.
- Prevention:
  - **Pre-exposure HDCV vaccination** for anyone who may be at risk for contact with infected animals. Three doses gives protection for 2 years.
  - **Vaccination of domestic and farm animals.**

Family: PARAMYXOVIVIRUS

GENERA AND SPECIES:	GENOME:
Paramyxovirus:	**ss(-) linear RNA**
Mumps: **F, H, N proteins**	
Parainfluenza: **F, H, N proteins**	
Morbillivirus:	SEGMENTATION:
Measles (Rubeola): **F, H proteins**	No other segments
Pneumovirus:	
Respiratory Syncytial virus:	NUCLEOCAPSID:
F-protein only	**Helical**

LOCATION OF REPLICATION:	ENVELOPE:
Cytoplasm	**Envelope**
EFFECT ON HOST CELL:	**F-,H-, N- proteins**
Buds from plasma membrane.	
No host cell lysis.	

SPECIAL FACTS:
F-protein: Fusion protein: enables fusion with host cells.
H-protein: Hemagglutinin: enhances attachment to host cells.
N-protein: Neuraminidase: breaks down neuraminic acid of mucus.

PATHOGENESIS:
Horizontal transmission is via **respiratory** route. In general, the upper respiratory tract and bronchial mucus membranes become infected. Both Measles and Mumps progress to viremia.

Genus: Paramyxovirus

Species: Mumps F, H, N: (only one type)
- **Disease: Mumps:**
  - **Parotitis:** painful swelling of parotid glands with fever; symptoms last about 2 weeks.
  - **Orchitis:** painful unilateral swelling of testes. (Sterility results from bilateral infection.)
  - **Aseptic Meningitis:** #1 cause of meningitis among non-immunized patients.
  - Self-limited symptoms; more severe in adults.
- **Transmission: respiratory** route, viremia, mostly **children**.
- **Geographic Range: World-wide.**
- **Diagnosis:** clinical presentation, serology.
- **Treatment:** symptom relief.
- **Immunity:** post-infectious, long-lasting immunity (IgG).
- **Vaccine: Live virus:** as part of **MMR** vaccine.
- Note: Vaccine may cause disease in immunocompromised: if given to compromised patient or to children in the household who may shed the virus after vaccination. However, MMR is given in **HIV** infected patients.

Species: Parainfluenza F, H, N: (many types)
- **Disease:**
  - **Croup (Laryngotracheobronchitis):** Characteristic cough.
  - **Upper Respiratory Tract Infections (URIs):** Otitis media, pharyngitis, common cold.
  - **Atypical Pneumonia.**
- **Transmission: respiratory** route, mostly **young children. Autumn** season.
- **Geographic Range: World-wide.**
- **Diagnosis:** clinical presentation, cell culture, and serology.
- **Treatment:** symptom relief.
- **Immunity:** post-infectious, type-specific immunity (IgG).
- **Vaccine:** none.

Genus: Morbillivirus

Species: Measles (Rubeola) F, H: (only one type)
- **Disease: Measles:** cough, **high fever** and **Koplik spots** (red spots with gray center, seen on buccal mucosa). **Rash** on **face first**, spreads to trunk and extremities. Measles virus is **highly contagious**.
  - **Atypical Pneumonia:** in **immunocompromised**, can be **fatal**.
  - **Encephalitis** and other **complications** occur.
- **Transmission: respiratory** route, viremia; mostly **children**.
- **Diagnosis:** clinical presentation, **Koplik spots**, serology
- **Treatment:** symptom relief. Immunocompromised patients need passive immunization with immunoglobulin.
- **Immunity:** post-infectious, long-lasting immunity (IgG).
- **Vaccine: Live virus:** as part of **MMR** vaccine.
- Note: Vaccine may cause disease in immunocompromised: if given to compromised patient or to children in the household who may shed the virus after vaccination. However, MMR is given in **HIV** infected patients.

Genus: Pneumovirus

Species: Respiratory Syncytial Virus F
- **Disease: Bronchiolitis-Pneumonia:** RSV is **most common** cause of lower respiratory tract infection in **infants**: wheezing, narrow bronchioles, air trapped in lungs (seen on X-ray).
  - **Upper Respiratory Tract Infections (URIs):**
- **Transmission: respiratory** route, mostly **infants** (< 6 mos), children and adults can get URI. **Winter** season.
- **Geographic Range: World-wide.**
- **Diagnosis:** clinical presentation, cell culture.
- **Treatment:** intense supportive care; **Ribavirin** (rarely used)
- **Immunity: reinfection** occurs due to incomplete immunity and **antigenic variation**.
- **Vaccine:** none.

Family: ORTHOMYXOVIRUS

GENERA AND SPECIES:

Influenza A virus:
Many antigenic subtypes based on **H-** and **N-** envelope protein spike combinations.
Influenza B virus:
Influenza C virus:

GENOME:
ss(-) linear RNA

SEGMENTATION:
8 RNA segments

NUCLEOCAPSID:
Helical

LOCATION OF REPLICATION:
Unique non-Retrovirus **RNA virus** to replicate in host cell

ENVELOPE:
Envelope
H-, N-proteins

EFFECT ON HOST CELL:
Buds from plasma membrane.
No host cell lysis.

SPECIAL FACTS:
- **H-protein:** Hemagglutinin: enhances attachment to host cells.
- **N-protein:** Neuraminidase: breaks down neuraminic acid of mucus.
NOTE: H-protein occurs in 3 types: H1, H2, H3.
       N-protein occurs in 3 types: N1, N2, N3.
- Viral types are represented by which protein combinations they have.
     Example: Influenza A/H3N2
- Epidemic types may be further categorized by city and year.
     Example: Influenza A/Singapore/86/H1N1
- **Antigenic Variation:**
    - **Antigenic Drift:** indicates a change in surface antigenic proteins due to minor **random mutations**. Does not lead to epidemics.
    - **Antigenic Shift:** indicates a change in surface antigenic proteins due to **resortment of RNA segments**. Only in Influenza A, and may lead to **epidemics** or **pandemics**.

PATHOGENESIS:
Horizontal transmission is via **respiratory** route. In general, the upper respiratory tract and bronchial mucus membranes and **ciliated** epithelial cells become infected and disrupted.

Genus: Influenza A

Species: Influenza A (many types)
- Disease:
    - **Influenza ("flu"):** constitutional symptoms: fever, chills, headache, myalgia and cough for 3 days.
    - **Atypical Pneumonia:** can be rapidly **fatal**.
    - **Secondary Bacterial Pneumonia:** destruction of respiratory cilia by initial flu infection enhances infection by *S. aureus* and other bacteria such as *S. pneumoniae*, and *H. influenzae*. Can be **fatal**.
    - **Reye Syndrome:** CNS complications may arise in **children** during infection by Influenza, especially if given **aspirin**. Can cause **seizures** and coma. Mostly **fatal**.
- **Special Outbreaks:**
    - **Endemic:** Influenza A infection has a world-wide baseline prevalence at all times.
    - **Epidemic:** Influenza A experiences sudden outbreaks above the base line, but restricted to one **region**.
    - **Pandemic:** Influenza A experiences sudden outbreaks above base line that spread across the **whole world**. Due to **Antigenic Shift**.
- **Antigenic Shift:**
    - Influenza A has the ability to generate new combinations of surface glycoproteins (H and N).
- Transmission: **respiratory** route, viremia. **Winter** season.
- Geographic Range: **World-wide**.
- Diagnosis: clinical presentation, virus isolation, serology.
- Treatment:
    - Symptomatic relief for mild cases.
    - **Amantadine** or **Rimantadine** in complicated cases
    - Antibiotics for cases of 2° bacterial pneumonia.
    - **Aspirin** must **NEVER** be given.
- Immunity: post-infectious, type-specific immunity (IgG).
- Vaccine: **dead virus:** new annual vaccine **every autumn**.

Genus: Influenza B

Species: Influenza B (many types)
- Disease:
    - **Influenza ("flu"):** constitutional symptoms: fever, chills, headache, myalgia and cough for 3 days.
    - **Atypical Pneumonia:** can be rapidly **fatal**.
    - **Secondary Bacterial Pneumonia:** can be **fatal**.
    - **Reye Syndrome:** CNS complications may arise in **children** during Influenza infection, especially if given **aspirin**. Can cause **seizures** and coma. Mostly **fatal**.
- **Special Outbreaks:**
- **Endemic:** Influenza B infection has a world-wide baseline prevalence at all times.
- **Epidemic:** Influenza B experiences sudden outbreaks above the base line, but restricted to one **region**.
- **Note:** Influenza B does **not** cause pandemics.
- Transmission: **respiratory** route, viremia. **Winter** season.
- Geographic Range: **World-wide**.
- Diagnosis: clinical presentation, virus isolation, serology.
- Treatment:
    - Symptomatic relief for mild cases.
    - Antibiotics for cases of 2° bacterial pneumonia.
    - **Aspirin** must **NEVER** be given.
- Immunity: post-infectious, type-specific immunity (IgG).
- Vaccine: **dead virus:** new annual vaccine **every autumn**.

Genus: Influenza C

Species: Influenza C
- Disease: minor respiratory illness.
- No epidemics; possible due to no antigenic variation.
- No treatment, self-limited.
- No vaccine.

Family: ARENAVIRUS

GENERA AND SPECIES:
Lymphocytic
Choriomeningitis:
Lassa Fever virus:

GENOME:
ss(-) Circular RNA

SEGMENTATION:
2 RNA segments
End to end to form a circle

NUCLEOCAPSID:
Helical

LOCATION OF REPLICATION:
Cytoplasm

ENVELOPE:
Envelope

EFFECT ON HOST CELL:
Buds from plasma membrane.
No host cell lysis.

SPECIAL FACTS:
● Arena = "Sandy," refers to ribosomes on the inner surface of envelope.
● Note: very unique RNA structure sometimes called "Ambisense" due to the way proteins are translated.

Genus: Lymphocytic Choriomeningitis Virus

Species: Lymphocytic Choriomeningitis Virus
● Disease:
  ▪ **Aseptic Meningitis:** CNS infection with high fever, headache, and myalgia; often self-limited.
  ▪ **LCV** infection during **pregnancy** results in fetal chorioretinitis (eye infection) and hydrocephalus.
  ▪ **Complications:** orchitis, myocarditis, arthritis.
● Transmission:
  ▪ **Zoonotic** transmission is via human contact with **rodent feces** or **urine** infected with virus:
      Reservoir = mice
      Host = human by contact with mice excrement
● Geographic Range: **N. America, S. America, Europe.**
● Diagnosis: virus isolation from blood and CSF.
● Treatment: supportive care.
● Immunity: post-infectious, type-specific immunity (IgG).
● Vaccine: none.

Genus: Lassa Fever Virus

Species: Lassa Fever Virus
● Disease:
  ▪ **Lassa Fever:** symptoms: **fever**, sore throat, myalgia, GI tract **bleeding**. Can progress to increased capillary permeability, multiorgan dysfunction and **shock**.
  Can be **fatal,** especially in **children**, but is often mild and self-limited.
  ▪ **Lassa Fever Virus** infection during **pregnancy** results in **abortion** and is often **fatal** to the mother.
● Transmission:
  ▪ **Zoonotic** transmission is via human contact with **rodent aerosols, feces** or **urine** infected with virus:
      Reservoir = mice
      Host = human by contact with mice excrement or mice aerosols.
  ▪ **Laboratory workers** may get infected while handling specimens
  ▪ **Horizontal** transmission from person to person occurs.
● Geographic Range: **West Africa.**
● Diagnosis:
  ▪ Virus isolation from blood and CSF.
  ▪ Serology.
  ▪ Elevated AST enzyme correlates to poor prognosis.
● Treatment: supportive care; **IV Ribavirin**.
● Immunity: post-infectious, type-specific immunity (IgG).
● Vaccine: none.

Family: RETROVIRUS

GENERA AND SPECIES:

Oncovirus Type C:
Human T-Cell Lymphotrophic Virus Type 1
Human T-Cell Lymphotrophic Virus Type 2
Lentivirus:
Human Immunodeficiency Virus Type 1
Human Immunodeficiency Virus Type 2
Spumavirus:
Human Foamy Virus

GENOME:
ss+ linear RNA
DIPLOID
Not Infectious RNA

SEGMENTATION:
2 RNA strands

NUCLEOCAPSID:
Complex

ENVELOPE:
Envelope

Note: Retrovirus RNA is **not** infectious because it does **not** encode RNA polymerase which can directly produce new RNA.

NOTE: HIV is presented on the next two pages.

HTLV GENES AND THE PROTEINS THEY ENCODE:

GAG Antigen Proteins: Used in packaging of virion core contents:
Capsid and **core** proteins.

POL Enzyme Proteins:
Protease: cleaves gag and pol coded proteins from precursors.
Reverse Transcriptase: RNA-dependent DNA-polymerase with RNAase activity to destroy RNA template.
Integrase: splices the proviral DNA into the host-cell genome.

ENV Antigen Glycoproteins:
Envelope surface and transmembrane glycoproteins.
Involved in attachment of virus to host cells.

TAX Promoter Protein:
Transactivation of both **viral** and **host** DNA **transcription**.

REX Regulation and Transport Protein:
Regulates RNA splicing; Transports mRNA out of nucleus.

LTR Long Terminal Repeats: promoter and enhancer regions.

HTLV UNIQUE EFFECT ON HOST CELL:
Buds from plasma membrane of **CD4+ T-cells**,
but causes T-cell **PROLIFERATION**, and not cell lysis.

Genus: Oncovirus

Species: HTLV-I
(Human T-Cell Lymphotrophic Virus Type 1)

- Disease:
  - **Adult T-Cell Leukemia/Lymphoma:**
  Malignant proliferation of **mature T-cells**; generalized lymphadenopathy, hepatosplenomegaly, and widespread cutaneous papulo-nodular lesions.
    - **Complications** are common due to impaired immunity: **Opportunistic** infections such as *Pneumocystis carinii* pneumonia, **fungal** infections, **Herpes virus** infections.
  - **Tropical Spastic Paraparesis:**
  Bilateral progressive weakness of lower limbs with some stiffness and some sensory loss. Hyperactive reflexes.
- Pathogenesis: the **hallmarks** of infection by HTLV-I are:
  1. Mostly **mature CD4+ T-cells** are infected.
  2. Infection causes **PROLIFERATION** of these T-cells.
- Transmission:
  - **Horizontal male to female** via **sexual contact**.
    (Virus is present in semen.)
  - **Horizontal male to male** via **homosexual contact**.
  - **Horizontal** via **IV drug abuse**, sharing needles.
  - **Iatrogenic** via **Blood transfusions**, organ transplants, and artificial insemination.
  - **Vertical mother to child** via **breast milk**.
    (No transplacental infection occurs.)
- Latency: up to **30-40 years**.
- Geographic Range: **Japan, S.E. USA, Caribbean, S. America,** and major cities worldwide.
- Diagnosis:
  - **Serology** test for **HTLV-I specific antibody**.
  - **Peripheral blood smear** shows atypical lymphocytes.
  - Presence of HTLV-I **provirus** in leukemic cells.
  - Elevated WBC as high as 100,000 cells/mm³
- Treatment: lymphoma chemotherapy.
- Vaccine: none.

Species: HTLV-II
(Human T-Cell Lymphotrophic Virus Type 2)

- Disease:
  - **Hairy Cell Leukemia:**
  HTLV-II infection is associated with this disease.
- Pathogenesis: similar to HTLV-I infection.
- Transmission:
  - **Horizontal male to female** via **sexual contact**.
    (Virus is present in semen.)
  - **Horizontal male to male** via **homosexual contact**.
  - **Horizontal** via **IV drug abuse**, sharing needles.
  - **Iatrogenic** via **Blood transfusions**, organ transplants, and artificial insemination.
  - **Vertical mother to child** via **breast milk**.
    (No transplacental infection occurs.)
- Latency: long time; unknown.
- Geographic Range: **Worldwide.**
- Diagnosis:
  - **Serology** test for **HTLV-II specific antibody**.
- Treatment:
- Vaccine: none.

RETROVIRUS continues on the next page.

Family: RETROVIRUS (cont'd)

Genus: Lentivirus

Convention of CD4 notation:
- CD4 or CD4+ or CD4 POS is used to designate a host cell which possesses the surface marker "CD4" (most often helper T-cells).
- CD4(-) or CD4 NEG likewise is used to indicate a host cell which does not possess the surface marker CD4.
- **"CD4 Count"** refers to the number of CD4+ cells per mm³ blood. The CD4 count in HIV infection shows a **characteristic pattern:** it decreases rapidly upon initial infection, rapidly returns to normal, then gradually and irreversibly declines over many years.

HIV EFFECT ON HOST CELL:
- **Buds** from plasma membrane of CD4 T-cells: causes **cell lysis** and **CD4 T-cell depletion.**

SPECIAL FACTS:
- HIV has a powerful ability to **rapidly mutate** due to the highly error-prone reverse transcriptase enzyme. This generates a widely variable **genetic diversity**, especially among its **envelope antigens**. This ability renders potential vaccines and antigen-targeted antiviral medications immediately ineffective. This ability also enables HIV to escape host immune responses.
- HIV is a highly **inefficient** virus due to the **error-prone enzymes** reverse transcriptase and integrase. Mostly non-functioning virions are generated. This handicap is overcome by HIV's **prolific nature**.
- HIV has the ability to **infect quiescent T-cells and Active T-cells**.
- HIV also has the ability to remain **latent** in host cells either in a **pre-integrated state** or in an **integrated state** (see life cycle step 8). Time of latency can vary from months to many years.

HIV GENES AND THE PROTEINS THEY ENCODE:

GAG Antigen Proteins: Involved in packaging of virion core contents: [Capsid protein: **p7**.] [Core proteins: **p24** and others.]

POL Enzyme Proteins:
- **Protease**: cleaves GAG and POL coded proteins from precursors.
- **Reverse Transcriptase**: RNA-dependent DNA-polymerase with **RNAase** activity to destroy RNA template..
- **Integrase**: inserts the proviral DNA into the host-cell genome.

ENV Antigen Glycoproteins: (precursor gp160 gets cleaved)
- **Envelope surface** glycoprotein: **gp120**
  - Involved in attachment of HIV to host cells such as **CD4+ T-cells** and **CD4+ Macrophages**.
  - **Connected to gp 41** on the virion surface.
- **Envelope transmembrane** glycoprotein: **gp41**
  - Involved in attachment of HIV to CD4(-) host cells such as glial cells and fibroblasts.
  - Enhances fusion of HIV to host cells after gp120 binds.
  - Enables fusion of host cells to form a **syncytium** wherein the virus will be better protected.

NOTE: gp120 and gp41 coding regions **mutate** easily and often, this enables HIV to escape antibodies and to thwart vaccines.

TAT Promoter Protein:
- **Transactivation** of HIV DNA **reverse transcription** increases HIV transcription 1000 fold.
- **Transactivation** of Host DNA **transcription** may promote transformation of proto-oncogenes into **oncogenes**.

REV Regulation and Transport Protein:
- Regulates RNA splicing; Transports mRNA out of nucleus.

NEF Negative Early Factor: promotes **latency** of HIV

VIF Virus Infectivity Factor: **anti-latency** gene of HIV
- Initiates replication, assembly, budding, and maturation.

VPR Transactivator.

VPU Stimulates virus release.

LTR Long Terminal Repeats: promoter and enhancer regions.
- **5' terminus LTR:** site of transcription activation and TAT binding

● Life cycle:

1. HIV gp120 attaches to **CD4** portion of **T-cells** and Macrophages. Note: HIV can also infect CD4 NEG cells, but the effect is unknown.
2. **Fusion** of HIV envelope with host cell membrane.
3. The HIV virion **core is released** into the host cell cytoplasm.
4. **Uncoating** of nucleocapsid enables release of GAG and POL proteins along with the HIV **genome**.
5. The HIV enzyme **Reverse transcriptase** initiates creation of the double-stranded "**proviral**" DNA from retroviral RNA.
6. **Retroviral RNA gets destroyed** by viral RNase.
7. Proviral DNA enters the nucleus.
8. The HIV enzyme **Integrase** integrates proviral DNA **randomly** into host cell genome. **Note:** HIV can remain **latent** in the host cell **either in the pre-integrated state or in the integrated state**.
9. Integrated proviral DNA is **transcribed** along with host cell DNA to generate RNA **by host RNA polymerase**.
10. This RNA is **translated** to proteins **by host ribosomes**.
11. HIV **envelope proteins** get **inserted in host plasma membrane**.
12. HIV **Capsid protein p7** begins **assembly** around the new HIV **genomic RNA dimer**, this takes place in the host cell cytoplasm.
13. HIV **virion buds through the host cell plasma membrane**.
14. This often causes **cell lysis**.
15. The **protease enzyme** begins its action at this point to **cleave** the newly translated precursor proteins into their functional components (see GAG and POL). This sets the stage for maturation.
16. **Maturation** is the **process of assembling the complex capsid**. Maturation occurs only after HIV budding and host cell lysis occur, and only after protease has successfully completed cleavage.

Note: this is an overview of the life cycle as it is currently proposed, these details are constantly being investigated and updated.

RETROVIRUS continues on the next page.

Family: RETROVIRUS (cont'd)

Please see previous page for **HIV gene products** and **HIV life cycle**.

NOTE: HIV is the **number one killer of men 25-44** in the USA; and the **number four killer of women 25-44** in the USA.
NOTE: AIDS as defined by the **CDC**= symptomatic HIV infection with a concurrent **CD4 count less than 200/mm³**
NOTE: VIRAL LOAD is measured by Plasma HIV RNA copies: Typical values are less than 20,000 copies per ml.

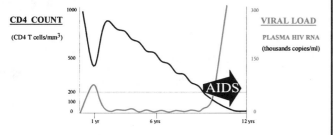

CD4 COUNT
(CD4 T cells/mm³)

VIRAL LOAD
PLASMA HIV RNA
(thousands copies/ml)

●Diagnosis:
SEROLOGY: (these tests may be negative for upto 6 mos).
▪**ELISA test: HIV surface gp120, gp160 specific antibody.**
▪**Western blot confirmation: HIV core p24, gp41 specific antibody.**
▪**Indirect Immunofluorescence Assay (IFA)** confirmation (p24,gp41)
OTHER:
▪**DNA probe with PCR** amplification to detect:
  -Proviral HIV DNA in peripheral mononuclear lymphocytes.
  -Replicating HIV RNA in plasma, to assess **"viral load."**
▪**Culture:** highly specific, but extremely insensitive. little value.
▪**ELISA test for Oral secretions:** very effective, needs confirmation.
▪**ELISA test for Urine:** not effective, no confirmation test available.
▪**Rapid ELISA for serum:** results in 10 min., needs confirmation.
▪**Home sample collection kits:** sent to lab, needs confirmation.

Genus: Lentivirus

Species: HIV-II:
Similar to HIV-I but causes less severe disease.

Species: HIV-I (Human Immunodeficiency Virus Type 1)
●Disease:
▪**Acute HIV infection:** initial presentation is with rash and fever but may be asymptomatic. Serology is negative.
▪**AIDS (Acquired Immune Deficiency Syndrome):**
Due to the severe, prolonged, and progressive drop in T-cell count, the T-cell mediated immunity becomes compromised. Relentless and invariably **fatal complications** begin.
●Complications:
▪**Wasting** and **chronic fatigue** may occur at any time, can be fatal.
▪**Malignancies:** especially **Kaposi's Sarcoma** and **Lymphomas.**
▪**AIDS-related dementia:** HIV encephalopathy at CD4 <200
▪**Opportunistic infections:**
  CD4 >200: *M. tuberculosis*, HSV , VZV .
  CD4 <200: *Candida* , *Pneumocystis carinii* **pneumonia,**
    Cryptococcus neoformans **meningitis.**
  CD4 <100: MAI **infection,** *N. asteroides* **infection,**
    Toxoplasma gondii **CNS infection.**
  CD4 <50: CMV **retinitis,** JC virus **PML.**
▪**Other infections:** Bacteria: *Bartonella, T. pallidum, salmonella.*
  Fungi: *C. immitis, H. capsulatum,*
  Protozoa: Amebas, *Cryptosporidium, Isospora.*
●Transmission:
  ▪**Horizontal via sexual contact:**
    HIV is present in semen and vaginal secretions.
  ▪**Horizontal** via **IV drug abuse,** sharing needles.
  ▪**Horizontal** : patient to **health care worker** via needle stick.
  ▪**Iatrogenic** via **Blood transfusions, organ transplants,** etc.
  ▪**Vertical** mother to child: **transplacentally in utero**
    or post-partum via **breast milk** .
●Geographic Range: **Worldwide.**

●Treatment: **Anti-retroviral medications:**
▪Nucleoside Anologues: **Zidovudine** (AZT, ZDV), **Didanosine** (ddI), **Zalcitabine** (ddC), **Lamivudine** (3TC), **Stavudine** (d4T)
  Mechanism of action:
  Inhibition of reverse transcriptase.
  DNA synthesis chain termination.
▪Protease inhibitors: **Indinavir, Nelfinavir, Ritinavir, Saquinavir.**
  Mechanism of action (⇩viral load and ⇧ CD4 count):
  Inhibition of protease enzyme: prevents cleavage of protein precursor products of GAG and POL genes. This stops viral maturation, and stops viral spread to other cells.
●Management:
Focus is on reduction of viral load, elevation of CD4 count, and on prevention or treatment of opportunistic infections. Prophylaxis and treatments must be **continued for life** because relapses usually occur.
▪**Emotional and educational support** is extremely important.
▪**Prophylaxis and treatment of HIV and opportunistic infections:**
  ▪*M. tuberculosis* prophylaxis: **Isoniazid** (INH).
  ▪At **CD4=500** begin double ℞: **AZT** plus **Indinavir.**
    Or triple ℞: **AZT**, plus **3TC**, plus **Indinavir.**
  ▪Upon failure of AZT: add or switch to **ddI** or **ddC.**
  ▪At **CD4=200** begin PCP prophylaxis: **TMP-SMZ.**
    Candida prophylaxis: **Fluconazole.**
  ▪At **CD4=100** begin MAI prophylaxis: **Rifabutin.**
    and *Toxoplasma* prophylaxis: **TMP-SMZ.**
  ▪At **CD4=50** CMV **retinitis** treatment.
▪**HIV in Pregnancy:** delivery by **cesarean section,** AZT for mother, **AZT** for newborn, **no breast feeding.**
●Vaccine: currently, there is no effective vaccine against HIV.
●Other helpful vaccines: **Hib** for H. influenzae; **Pneumovax** for S. pneumoniae; And **Influenza** virus vaccine.
▪It is necessary to **avoid live-organism vaccines** except MMR.
●Prevention: abstinence from risky sexual contact; use of condoms. Health care workers must use universal precautions.

Chapter 18

PRIONS   (Proteinaceous Infectious Particles)

PRIONS:

Non-DNA, Non-RNA, Protein particles:

●Prions cause **chronic**, latent, **slowly progressive**, and consistently **fatal** infections of the **CNS**. These infections are often called **"Slow Infections"** or "**Transmissible Neurodegenerative Diseases**."

●The CNS pathological changes are described as **non-inflammatory "spongiform" encephalopathy**; characterized by **"Swiss cheese-like" vacuoles** within brain parenchyma.

●Prions resist destruction by agents which destroy nucleic acids, but are destroyed by agents which destroy proteins.

●Prions infect neurons, spread through the CNS by axonal transport, and **replicate** by some unknown means. Very little is known about Prions.

●The normal human **PrP gene** codes for a normal protein, designated **PrPc**. Prion protein is similar to this protein. However, Prion protein, designated **PrPsc**, is not a gene-product of the human PrP gene.

●Disease: **CREUTZFELDT-JAKOB DISEASE**
▪Very **rare** disease usually begins in middle age.
▪Disease is manifest by variable neurological symptoms, invariably myoclonus, and rapidly progressive **dementia**.
▪Seizures are rare, cranial nerve involvement is rare.
▪**Rapidly fatal** within months.
●Transmission:
▪**Horizontal** transmission occurs rarely.
▪**Iatrogenic** infection occurs due to use of contaminated surgical instruments; due to contaminated corneal transplants; or due to use of contaminated cadaver-derived human hormones.
▪**Familial**-autosomal dominant inheritance occurs.
●**Warnings:**
▪**Health care workers** may be at risk of infection while handling neural tissue and CSF, especially during **neurosurgery**, during **autopsy**, or during work with brains of **cadavers**.
▪Universal precautions and eye protection are recommended.
▪Instrument sterilization requires minimum of 1 hour autoclaving at 132°C or 1 hour immersion in 1 N Na OH
●Diagnosis:
▪CT scan, MRI and CSF may be normal.
▪EEG is usually abnormal.
▪Brain biopsy shows **spongiform change** with **no inflammation**.
▪Immunostaining of brain reveals **PrPsc** protein **infectious particle**.
●Treatment: **None**.

●Disease: **KURU**
▪Very rare disease limited to one tribal group of Papua-New Guinea.
▪Disease is mostly characterized by cerebellar ataxia, intentional tremors, myoclonic jerks, and choreoathetoid movements.
▪Fatal within months-years.
●Transmission:
▪**Horizontal** transmission occurs via **cannibalistic ingestion** of infected human brains, and via **handling** of infected human brains.
▪Limited to Papua-New Guinea.
●Diagnosis:
▪Brain biopsy shows **spongiform change** with **no inflammation**.
▪Immunostaining of brain reveals **PrPsc** protein **infectious particle**.
●Treatment: **None**.

●Disease: **FAMILIAL PRION DISEASES:**
▪**Familial Fatal Insomnia**.
▪**Gerstmann-Straussler-Scheinker Syndrome**.
▪**Familial Creutzfeldt-Jakob Disease**.
●Diagnosis:
▪Brain biopsy shows **spongiform change** with **no inflammation**.
▪Immunostaining of brain reveals **PrPsc** protein as a product of the **mutated PrP gene**.
●Treatment: **None**.

Chapter 19

VIRUS CROSS REFERENCE (Part 1)

BUDS FROM NUCLEUS
Herpesviruses

**ONLY DNA VIRUS TO
REPLICATE IN CYTOPLASM**
Poxvirus

SMALLEST VIRUS
Parvovirus

LARGEST VIRUS
Poxvirus

"INFECTIOUS" VIRUSES
[ss+ RNA genome]
[Encode RNA polymerase]
    Picornaviruses
    Caliciviruses
    Togaviruses
    Flaviviruses
    Coronaviruses

DIPLOID RNA
Retroviruses

**RNA VIRUSES WHICH
REPLICATE IN NUCLEUS**
Orthomyxoviruses
Retroviruses

NO ECLIPSE PERIOD
Reoviruses

"SLOW VIRUS" INFECTIONS

JC virus Latent infection:
**Progressive Multifocal
    Leukoencephalopathy** (PML)

Measles virus Latent infection:
**Subacute Sclerosing
    PanEncephalitis** (SSPE)

Retroviruses:
    HTLV-1 Latent as
T-cell Leukemia/Lymphoma or as
Tropical Spastic Paraparesis (TSP)
    HTLV-2 Possibly latent as
Hairy Cell Leukemia
    HIV Latent infection:
**Acquired Immuno-Deficiency
    Syndrome** (AIDS)

PRION SLOW INFECTIONS
Creutzfeldt-Jakob Disease
Kuru
Familial Fatal Insomnia
Gerstmann-Straussler-Scheinker
    Syndrome

**ARBOVIRUSES
(vector-borne)**
Togaviruses (except Rubivirus)
Flaviviruses (except Hepatitis C)
Reovirus coltivirus
Bunyaviruses

HEPATITIS VIRUSES

Picornavirus Hepatitis A
    Acute Hepatitis

Calicivirus Hepatitis E
    Acute Hepatitis

Flavivirus Hepatitis C
Blood-transfusion hepatitis
    Acute Hepatitis
    Chronic Hepatitis
    Carrier State Hepatitis

Hepadnavirus Hepatitis B
Sexually-transmitted hepatitis
    Acute Hepatitis
    Chronic Hepatitis
    Carrier State Hepatitis
    Fulminant Hepatitis

Defective virus Hepatitis D
[Requires HBV infection]
    Acute Hepatitis
    Chronic Hepatitis
    Carrier State Hepatitis
    Fulminant Hepatitis

VIRUS CROSS REFERENCE (Part 2)

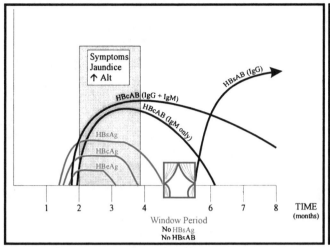

Hepatitis B Infection

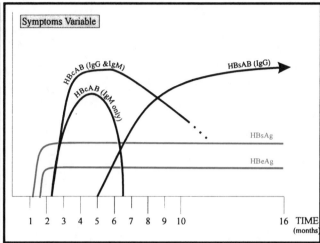

Hepatitis B Transmissible Carrier

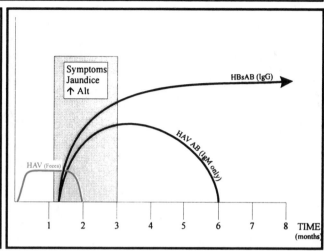

Hepatitis A Infection

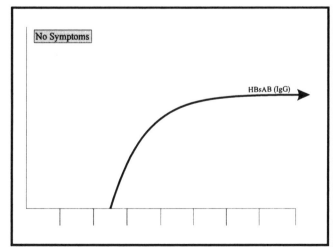

Hepatitis B Immunization

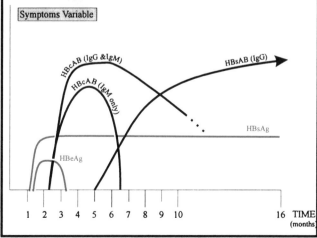

Hepatitis B Non-Transmissible Carrier

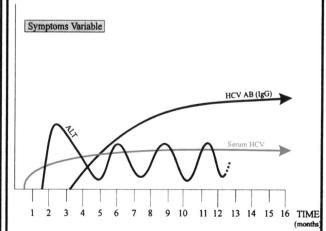

Hepatitis C Infection

Chapter 20

FUNGI: MYCOTIC DISEASE (MYCOSIS)

Fungus: Eukaryotic; Cell wall of chitin; Cell membrane of ergosterol.
Yeast: Fungal single cell phase.
Mold (mycelial): Fungal multicellular filamentous colony phase.
Dimorphic: when a fungal species can exist in yeast phase or mold phase depending on environmental conditions.

Category: **CUTANEOUS FUNGI**
Route of Infection: **Contact or Trauma**
Organisms:

Dermatophytes:
Epidermophyton spp
Microsporum spp
Trichophyton spp
- Tinea (ring worm)

Superficials:
Exophiala werneckii
- Tinea Nigra
(brown spots)
Malassezia furfur
- Pityriasis Versicolor
(hypopigmentation)
- **DIMORPHIC**
Piedraia hortae
- Black Piedra
(black nodules on scalp hair roots)
Trichosporon cutaneum
- White Piedra
(yellow nodules on axilla, beard and groin hair shafts)

Category: **SUBCUTANEOUS FUNGI**
Route of Infection: **Trauma**
Organisms:

Sporothrix schenckii
- Ulcerative lymphatic tracts
- From thorns
- **DIMORPHIC**

Cladosporium spp
Fonsecaea spp
Phialophora spp
- Chromomycosis
(wart-like granulomas of feet, legs)

Madurella spp
Pseudallescheria spp
- Mycetoma
(abscesses and sinus tracts of feet)

Category: **SYSTEMIC FUNGI**
Route of Infection: **Respiratory**
Organisms:

Blastomyces dermatitidis
- Pulmonary infection
- Granulomatous ulcers of skin and bone
- **DIMORPHIC**

Coccidioides immitis
- Pulmonary infection
- Erythema Nodosum
("Valley fever," "desert rheumatism")
- **DIMORPHIC**

Histoplasma capsulatum
- Pulmonary infection, pneumonia
- **DIMORPHIC**

Paracoccidioides brasiliensis
- Pulmonary infection
- **DIMORPHIC**

Category: **OPPORTUNISTIC FUNGI**
Route of Infection: **Colonization during immunocomromised state**
Organisms:

Aspergillus fumigatus
Aspergillus flavus
- Fungus balls in lungs
- Chronic sinusitis
- Allergic Asthma
- *Aspergillus flavus* produces **Aflatoxin**.
Candida albicans
- Oral thrush
- Diaper rash
- Vaginitis
- Disseminated disease
Cryptococcus neoformans
- CNS infection, meningitis
(grows well in CSF)

Mucormycosis:
Absidia spp
Mucor spp
Rhizopus spp
- Paranasal sinus necrosis
- Especially in Diabetics

CUTANEOUS FUNGI

Dermatophytes: *Epidermophyton spp*
Microsporum spp
Trichophyton spp

●Diseases: **Tinea:** "ring worm," annular rash.
    Tinea capitis: scalp, hair-shaft infection.
        Mostly in children, highly **contagious**.
    Tinea barbae: beard infection.
    Tinea corporis: body infection.
    Tinea cruris: "jock -itch"
    Tinea pedis: "athlete's foot"
    Onychomycosis: finger/toe nail infection.
●Transmission: horizontal via direct contact; especially in warm, damp conditions. Dermatophytes are nurtured by keratin in skin. *Microsporum* are found on dogs and cats.
●Diagnosis:
▪Skin/hair/nail **scrapings** preserved in **10%KOH** examined to see **mold** form **septated hypae**.
▪Scrapings may be cultured on **Sabouraud agar**.
▪**Wood's Lamp:** green fluorescence of *Microsporum* hair.
●Treatment:
    ▪**Topical antifungals**.
    ▪**Griseofulvin** (oral)
        for Tinea Capitis and Onychomycosis.
    ▪Keep skin cool and dry.

Exophiala werneckii

●Disease: **Tinea Nigra:** brown spots on palms and soles.
●Transmission: infection arises due to direct contact,
    Exophiala is found in soil.
●Diagnosis:
    Skin scrapings/ microscopy show mold hyphae.
●Treatment:
    ▪Topical keratolytic agent.
    ▪Topical Salicylic acid

Malassezia furfur

(formerly *Pityrosporum ovale* and *Pityrosporum orbiculare*)

●Disease: **Pityriasis Versicolor (Tinea versicolor):**
    non-itchy, depigmenting lesions on shoulders,
    chest, back, upper arms.
●Transmission:
Malassezia furfur usually exist as **commensal yeast** on most human scalps. Disease arises when the **yeast phase** fungi **transform** into the **mold phase** fungi with **hyphae**. Cause of transformation is unknown.
●Diagnosis:
Skin scrapings preserved in **10%KOH** then microscopy show round **yeast forms** present along with **short hyphal mold forms**.
Note: **DIMORPHIC** (yeast and mold forms occur).
●Treatment:
    ▪Topical azole antifungal cream
    ▪Oral Ketoconazole
    ▪Often relapses

Piedraia hortae

●Disease: **Black Piedra:** black nodules on scalp hair roots.
●Transmission: horizontal via direct contact.
●Diagnosis: Skin scrapings/ microscopy show mold hyphae.
●Treatment:
    ▪Topical Salicylic acid.

Trichosporon cutaneum

●Disease: **White Piedra:** yellow nodules on axilla, beard and groin hair shafts.
●Transmission: horizontal via direct contact; sexual contact
●Diagnosis: Skin scrapings/ microscopy show mold hyphae.
●Treatment:
    ▪Oral Ketoconazole.
    ▪Relapse is expected.

SUBCUTANEOUS FUNGI

Sporothrix schenckii

●Disease: **Sporotrichosis:**
>painless nodules form along lymphatic channels, these nodules sometimes ulcerate.

●Transmission: infection arises due to puncture wounds or scratches while **gardening**; especially by rose bush **thorns**, wood **splinters**, hay, straw, or mosses.

●Diagnosis:
▪Skin tissue specimen preserved in **10%KOH** examined to see **"cigar-shaped" budding yeast**.
▪Skin tissue specimen may be **cultured** on **Sabouraud agar**, to grow the **mold form** which has characteristic **hyphae** with **"daisy" cluster of conidia**.

Note: **DIMORPHIC** (yeast and mold forms occur).

●Treatment:
>▪**Oral Potassium Iodide**

●Prevention:
>▪Wear protective clothing while gardening.

Cladosporium spp
Fonsecaea spp
Phialophora spp

●Disease: **Chromomycosis:** papular, verrucous, and sometimes pedunculated or cauliflower-like growths due to chronic infection of subcutaneous tissues. These growths develop slowly over years and show central clearing as they spread. No ulcerations or sinus tract formations occur. Feet and legs are the most common sites of infection.

●Transmission: infection arises due to puncture wound while working with **rotting wood** or soil.

●Diagnosis:
▪Skin scrapings preserved in **10%KOH** examined to see **brown "copper penny"** fungi in Macros .

●Treatment:
>▪Surgical excision.

Madurella spp
Pseudallescheria spp

●Disease: **Fungal Mycetoma (Eumycetoma):**
Abscess formation of subcutaneous tissues and bones with a pus-like discharge from multiple **sinus tracts** which form along lymphatic channels mostly on **feet**, sometimes on hands or elsewhere. The **pus** contains varied-**colored granules**.

●Transmission: infection arises due to puncture wound or trauma while walking with unprotected **feet** on **soil**.

●Diagnosis:
>Microscopy of pus shows **mold hyphae** and characteristic species-specific **colored granules**.

●Treatment:
>▪Combination of Dapsone,TMP-SMZ, and Surgery.

●Prevention:
>▪Wear shoes.

SYSTEMIC FUNGI

Blastomyces dermatitidis

- Disease: **Blastomycosis:** initial mild **pulmonary** infection spreads via **hematogenous route** to manifest as **verrucous** and **ulcerative skin lesions**.
- Transmission: infection arises due to **inhalation** of the **mold** conidia from **dust-clouds** at construction sites or **crop-dust** during harvesting on farms. Most common in the **Mississippi river valley**, the **mid-west** and **south** USA; occurs worldwide.
  Note: this is **not contagious**.
- Diagnosis:
- Skin tissue specimen or **sputum** preserved in **10%KOH** examined to see **multi-nucleated yeast** which undergo **single broad-based budding**.
- Skin tissue specimen may be **cultured** on Sabouraud agar, to grow the **mold form** which has characteristic **septated branching hyphae with microconidia**.
  Note: **DIMORPHIC** (yeast and mold forms occur).
- Treatment: **Itraconazole**

Coccidioides immitis

- Disease: **Coccidioidomycosis:**
  - **Influenza-like** pulmonary infection with fever, cough.
  - **Erythema Nodosum with Arthralgia:**
    "Valley Fever" and **"desert rheumatism"** (west USA) usually resolves spontaneously.
  - **Pneumonia** and disseminated disease. Can be **fatal**. May disseminate to bone, joints, skin or meninges. Disseminated disease is common in **AIDS** patients and **pregnant** women during **3rd trimester**.
- Transmission: infection arises due to **inhalation** of the **mold arthrospores** from **soil**. Most common in **warm climates** of the USA, Central America, and South America.
  Note: this is **not contagious**.
- Diagnosis:
- **Lung** or other **tissue specimen** or **sputum** preserved in **10%KOH**, stained with lactophenol cotton blue, examined to see **yeast "spherules"** which are round pouches that contain **endospores**, no budding.
- **Specimen** may be **cultured** on Sabouraud agar, to grow the **mold form** which has characteristic **septated branching hyphae with arthrospores**.
  Warning: culture-grown spores are **infectious** to lab personnel.
- **Serology:** IgM and IgG antibodies to mold phase antigens; or complement-fixing antibody titer (CF test).
- **Skin test** (turns NEG in chronic disease due to anergy)
- **Chest X-Ray:** calcifications, granulomas.
  Note: **DIMORPHIC** (yeast and mold forms occur).
- Treatment:
  Amphotericin B
  Fluconazole for meningitis.

Histoplasma capsulatum

- Disease: **Histoplasmosis:** very similar to **tuberculosis**; pneumonia, granulomas, and caseating necrosis may heal to form "coin lesion" (focal calcification). **Chronic** disease may lead to **cavitation** and **dissemination** in blood. Can be **fatal**.
- Transmission: infection arises due to **inhalation** of the **mold** conidia from **moist soil**, **bird droppings**, and **bat droppings**. Mostly in **central/eastern USA**; occurs worldwide.
- Diagnosis:
- **Lung tissue specimen or sputum** preserved in **10%KOH**, stained with silver or Giemsa stain, examined to see **oval yeast** which **undergo budding within Macros**.
- **Specimen** may be **cultured** on Sabouraud agar, to grow the **mold form** which has characteristic **septated branching hyphae** with **microconidia** and **turberculated macroconidia**.
  Warning: culture-grown spores are **infectious** to lab personnel.
- **Serology:** complement-fixating antibody titer (CF test).
- **DTH skin test** (turns NEG in chronic disease due to anergy)
- **Antigen Detection:** urine antigen, serum antigen.
- **Chest X-Ray:** calcifications, granulomas.
  Note: **DIMORPHIC** (yeast and mold forms occur).
- Treatment: **Itraconazole** or **Amphotericin B**

Paracoccidioides brasiliensis

- Disease: Pulmonary infection similar to tuberculosis; remains sub-clinical or dormant; progresses upon diminished immunity. Oral mucosal lesions also occur.
- Transmission: infection arises due to **inhalation** of **mold spores** from soil. Mostly in rural Central and South America.
- Diagnosis:
- **Lung tissue specimen or sputum** preserved in **10%KOH**, examined to see **yeast** which **undergo multiple budding**.
- **Sputum** may be **cultured** on Sabouraud agar to grow **mold**.
- **Serology** can be used to follow the disease.
  Note: **DIMORPHIC** (yeast and mold forms occur).
- Treatment: **Itraconazole**

OPPORTUNISTIC FUNGI

Aspergillus fumigatus
Aspergillus flavus

- Disease: **Aspergillosis:**
    - **Aspergilloma: "fungus balls in lung"**
        (fungus balls are groups of mold hyphae):
        Arise in patients with **pre-existing lung disease**
        (e.g. within an old tuberculosis cavity).
        Causes **hemoptysis**; can be **fatal**.
    - **Chronic sinusitis** of paranasal sinuses; may form
        "fungus balls" in sinuses.
    - **Allergic Asthma** from mold spores.
    - *A. flavus* produces **Aflatoxin** on nuts and grains.
        Aflatoxin is toxic and **carcinogenic**.
- Transmission: *Aspergillus* molds are ubiquitous in nature,
  especially in soil and decaying vegetation. Infection arises due to
  inhalation of **mold spores** while the host is **immunocompromised**.
- Diagnosis:
    - **Lung tissue specimen or sputum** preserved in **10%KOH**,
        examined to see **mold form** which has characteristic
        septated branching hyphae with **spores**.
    - **Specimen** may be **cultured** on Sabouraud agar.
    - **Chest X-Ray:** shows air pockets and evidence of fungus balls.
    Note: *Aspergillus* exist in **mold form only**, even when they invade
    tissues.
- Treatment:
    - **Surgery** for fungus balls.
    - **Amphotericin B**

Candida albicans

- Disease: **Candidiasis:**
    - **Oral Thrush:** focal **white** patches on oral mucosa and tongue;
        they **bleed** when scraped off.
    - **Cutaneous Candidiasis:** blotchy red, itchy rash which spreads
        and may occur anywhere. "Diaper Rash" in **infants**.
    - **Onychomycosis and Paronychia:** infection of finger/toe **nails**
        and **nail folds**; usually from chronic **wet hands** as from
        washing dishes, etc.
    - **Vaginitis:** very **common** infection among women. May be
        asymptomatic or yield a **curd-like discharge** and cause
        pruritus of vulva.
    - **Chronic Mucocutaneous Candidiasis:** disseminated disease
        may lead to chronic infections anywhere such as skin
        heart (endocarditis), lungs, CNS (meningitis), bone, etc.
- Transmission: Candida albicans is a normal **commensal** of human **GI**
  tract and **female genital** tract. Infection arises either due to **destruction** of
  other **host commensals** (as occurs during use of some **antibiotics**), or due
  to **immunocompromised** state of the host. Usually, candidiasis infections
  are not contagious.
- Diagnosis:
    - **Tissue specimen** preserved in **10%KOH**, examined to see **budding**
        yeast with **pseudohyphi**.
    - **Germ tubes**, unique to *C. albicans*, may be seen extending from round
        yeast forms; this is found in **serum** during disseminated disease.
    - **Specimens** may be **cultured** on Sabouraud agar to grow **yeast** which
        have **chlamydospores** (unique to *C. albicans*) and **blastospores**.
    - **Skin test:** POS in most people, will be NEG in immunocompromised
        patients to indicate anergy.
- Treatment:
    - **Clotrimazole:** oral lozenge.
    - **Nystatin:** oral, topical or suppository.
    - **Amphotericin B** for disseminated disease.

Cryptococcus neoformans

- Disease: **Cryptococcosis:**
    - **Pulmonary infection:** may be mild or severe and **fatal**.
    - **Meningitis:** *C. neoformans* disseminates rapidly from pulmonary
        infection then **thrives in CSF**. Meninges are diffusely infected,
        and infection spreads rapidly to brain parenchyma.
    Complications: Cranial nerve palsies, blindness, hydrocephalus, and
        cerebral edema. Can be **fatal**, relapse is common, persistence
        of neurological deficits is common. Incurable in **AIDS** patients.
- Transmission: *Cryptococcus* are ubiquitous in nature. Infection arises
  in **immunocompromised** patients due to inhalation of yeast from soil or
  from pigeon droppings.
- Diagnosis:
    - **CSF specimen** preserved in **10%KOH**, stained with **India Ink**,
        examined to see **encapsulated yeast** which undergo budding.
    - **Tissue specimens** may be stained with Mayer's mucicarmine stain:
        the large capsule, unique to *Cryptococcus*, will appear pink.
    - **Serology** to detect the capsular antigen.
    - **Urease test:** isolates show positve urease test within 15 min.
- Treatment: **Amphotericin B** plus **Flucytosine**.

Absidia spp
Mucor spp
Rhizopus spp

- Disease: **Mucormycosis:** (old terms: phycomycosis or zygomycosis):
  These fungi invade blood vessel walls: cause tissue necrosis; especially
  in **paranasal sinuses**, brain, lungs, and GI tract. Can be **fatal**.
- Transmission: these fungi are ubiquitous in nature, especially as bread
  molds. Infection is very rare and arises due to **immunocompromised**
  situations, especially in **diabetic** patients.
- Diagnosis:
    - **Tissue specimen** preserved in **10%KOH**, examined to see **mold** with
        non-septate hyphae which **branch at right angles**, and **sporangium**.
- Treatment:
    - **Surgery**
    - **Amphotericin B**

Chapter 21

FUNGI: CROSS REFERENCE

INTRACELLULAR
Cladosporium spp
Fonsecaea spp
Phialophora spp
Histoplasma capsulatum

INDIA INK STAIN
Cryptococcus neoformans

CHLAMYDOSPORES
Candida albicans

GERM TUBES
Candida albicans

DIMORPHIC
Malassezia furfur
Sporothrix schenckii
Blastomyces dermatitidis
Coccidioides immitis
Histoplasma capsulatum
Paracoccidioides brasiliensis

MOLD ONLY
Dermatophytes
　　　Epidermophyton spp
　　　Microsporum spp
　　　Trichophyton spp
Aspergillus fumigatus
Absidia spp
Mucor spp
Rhizopus spp

YEAST ONLY
Cryptococcus neoformans
Candida albicans

NON-SEPTATED HYPHI
Absidia spp
Mucor spp
Rhizopus spp

PSEUDO-HYPHI
Candida albicans

TOXIN PRODUCING
Aspergillus flavus (aflatoxin)

FOOTBALL-SHAPE CONIDIA
Microsporum spp

DAISY-SHAPED CONIDIA
Sporothrix schenckii

CIGAR-SHAPED YEAST
Sporothrix schenckii

MULTINUCLEATED YEAST
Blastomyces dermatitidis

SHERULE YEAST
Coccidioides immitis

MULTIPLE-BUDDING YEAST
Paracoccidioides brasiliensis

ENCAPSULED YEAST
Cryptococcus neoformans

ANIMAL-RELATED
Microsporum spp (cats, dogs)
Histoplasma capsulatum
　　　　　(birds, bats)
Cryptococcus neoformans
　　　　　(birds)

SKIN TESTS
Coccidioides immitis
Histoplasma capsulatum
Candida albicans

NOTE: 1. These light microscope color plates represent typical specimens(not ideal specimens) as encountered in clinical practice.
2. All of the color plates on this page are magnified to equal high power to allow meaningful comparison of relative sizes.

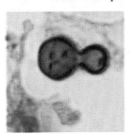

Blastomyces dermatitidis Budding.
Tissue biopsy (GMS stain)

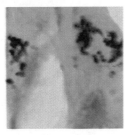

Coccidioides immitis Spherule.
Tissue biopsy (GMS stain)

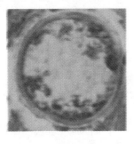

Histoplasma capsulatum
Tissue biopsy (GMS stain)

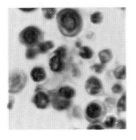

Candida albicans
Tissue biopsy (GMSstain)

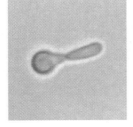

Candida albicans Germ tube.
Incubated in serum for 3 hours

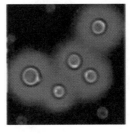

Cryptococcus neoformans with Capsules.
CSF (India Ink stain)

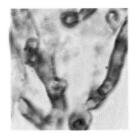

Aspergillus fumigatus
Tissue biopsy (GMS stain)

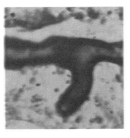

Mucor spp, Rhizopus spp
Tissue biopsy (GMS stain)

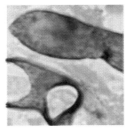

Mucor spp, Rhizopus spp
Tissue biopsy (GMS stain)

Chapter 22

PARASITES:

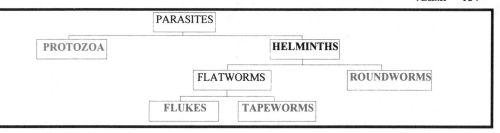

PROTOZOA:

PNEUMOCYSTIS:
Pneumocystis carinii Pneumonia

AMEBAS:
Entamoeba hystolytica Dysentery
Naegleria fowleri Meningoencephalitis
Acanthamoeba spp Meningoencephalitis
                                    Keratitis

FLAGELLATES:
Giardia lamblia Diarrhea
Trichomonas vaginalis Vaginal discharge
Leishmania donovani Kala-azar
Leishmania spp Oriental sore
Trypanosoma cruzi Chagas
Trypanosoma spp African sleeping sickness

SPOROZOANS:
Cryptosporidium spp Diarrhea
Isospora spp Diarrhea
Toxoplasma gondii Encephalitis
Plasmodium spp: Malaria
        P. falciparum
        P. malariae
        P. ovale
        P. vivax
Babesia spp Malaria-like illness

HELMINTH
FLAT WORM (Platyhelminth)
FLUKES: **TREMATODA**

SCHISTOSOMIASIS:
Schistosoma haematobium
Schistosoma japonicum
Schistosoma mansoni

LIVER FLUKE:
Clonorchis sinensis

LUNG FLUKE:
Paragonimus westermani

HELMINTH
FLAT WORM (Platyhelminth)
TAPE WORMS: **CESTODA**

PORK TAPEWORM and Cysticercosis:
Taenia solium

BEEF TAPEWORM:
Taenia saginata

FISH TAPEWORM:
Diphyllobothrium latum

HYDATID CYSTS:
Echinococcus granulosus
Echinococcus multilocularis

HELMINTH
ROUND WORMS: **NEMATODA**

INTESTINAL NEMATODES:
        [Humans as Intermediary Host]:
Ancylostoma duodenale Hook worm
Necator americanus Hook worm
Strongyloides stercoralis Thread worm

Ascaris lumbricoides Largest nematode
Enterobius vermicularis Pin worm
Trichuris trichiura Whip worm

EXTRAINTESTINAL LARVAE:
        [Humans as Dead-End Host]:
Ancylostoma caninum Cutaneous Larva Migrans
Toxocara canis Visceral Larva Migrans
Trichinella spiralis Trichinosis

TISSUE NEMATODES
        [Vector-Borne Larvae]:
Dirofilaria immitis (dog heart worm) Lung lesion
Loa loa Eye worm
Onchocerca volvulus River Blindness
Wuchereria bancrofti Filariasis, Elephantiasis
Brugia spp Filariasis, Elephantiasis
        [Non-Vector Larvae]:
Dracunculus medinensis Guinea worm

PROTOZOA   Just The Essentials.

PROTOZOA FEATURES:
- **Unicellular.**
- **Cyst** = non-motile, encapsulated, transmission stage in the life cycle.
- **Trophozoite** = motile, feeding, multiplying stage in the life cycle.

PNEUMOCYSTIS: (can be classified as yeast phase of fungus)
Pneumocystis carinii
- Disease: **Interstitial pneumonia**
    - *P. carinii* **Pneumonia** is known as **"PCP":**
    - Also called "Plasma Cell Pneumonia."
    - Occurs in **immunocompromised** patients.
    - Common in **AIDS** patients with **CD4 count < 200.**
- Infection: arises due to inhalation of *P. carinii* cysts.
    - The cysts and trophozoites cause interstitial inflamation.
    - *P. carinii* is ubiquitous in nature. Highly **fatal** in AIDS.
- Note: PCP is probably **not contagious.**
- Diagnosis: Bronchoscopy biopsy: silver stain shows **cysts.**
- Treatment and prophylaxis: **TMP-SMZ.**

AMEBAS:

Entamoeba hystolytica:
- Diseases: **Amebiasis:**
    - **Dysentery** with **bloody diarrhea:**
        - Invade colon to cause "tear-drop ulcer,"
        - no PMNs respond, no inflammation.
    - **Liver abscesses**
- Infection: *Entamoeba* **Cysts** via **fecal-oral** route.
    - **Cysts** mature in small intestine **lumen** to become
    - Trophozoites. **Trophozoites** invade colon and liver.
- Diagnosis:
    - **Cysts** found in solid stool. Serology confirmation.
    - **Trophozoites** found in diarrhea, they ingest RBCs.
    - **Ultrasound** for liver abscess.
- Treatment:
    - **Diloxanide fuoate** for **luminal** infection.
    - **Iodoquinol** in pregnancy for luminal.
    - **Metronidazole** for tissue invasion of colon or liver.

Naegleria fowleri
Acanthamoeba spp
- Diseases: **Meningoencephalitis; Keratitis**
- Infection:
    - **Meningoencephalitis** occurs via **swimming** in **warm fresh water** as the **trophozoites** enter nasal mucosa then pass cribriform plate. **Southern USA.**
- (Note: *Acanthamoeba* meningoencephalitis occurs only in immunocompromised patients.)
    - **Keratitis,** most often by *Acanthamoeba,* occurs mostly in healthy **contact lens users.**
- Treatment: **Amphotericin B** for CNS infection.
    - Propamidine isethionate for keratitis.

FLAGELLATES:

Giardia lamblia
- Disease: **Persistent Foul-smelling diarrhea,** no fever.
- Infection:
- **Fecal-oral** route: **Cysts** in contaminated water get ingested; undergo excystation in doudenum to become trophozoites; **Trophozoites** attach to intestinal wall.
    - **Horizontal transmission:**
        - Common among children and homosexuals.
    - **Zoonotic transmission:**
        - Common in hikers who drink stream water.
- Diagnosis: **Stool sample:**
    - **Cysts or trophozoites** with Trichrome stain.
    - Stool antigen detection kits are available.
- Treatment: **Metronidazole**
    - Prevention: Boil or Filter the water.

Leishmania donovani   ▪**Kala-azar** (visceral)
Leishmania spp   ▪**Oriental Sore** (cutaneous)
- Vector: **sand-fly**   ▪Treatment: Stibogluconate

Trichomonas vaginalis
- **Vaginitis:** Green, **foul-smelling vaginal discharge.**
- **Sexually-Transmitted Disease.**
- Diagnosis by wet-mount of discharge: trophozoites.
- Treatment: **Metronidazole** for patient and partner.

Trypanosoma cruzi
- **Chagas Disease:** *T. cruzi* invade cardiac myocytes to cause arrhythmias; invade nerve plexus of GI tract to cause **mega-colon** and mega-esophagus.
- Vector: **Reduviid Bug;**   ▪Treatment: Nifurtimox

Trypanosoma spp
- **African sleeping sickness:** fever, demyelinating encephalitis, coma. Ability to **alter surface antigens**
- Vector: **Tsetse-fly**   ▪Treatment: Suramin.

PROTOZOA
SPOROZOANS

Cryptosporidium spp
Isospora spp
●Diseases: **Diarrhea** in **immunocompromised**.
Note: *Cryptosporidiu* and *Isospora* stool sample smear shows **oocysts** as **Modified Acid Fast Stain**.

Toxoplasma gondii
●Diseases: **Toxoplasmosis:**
▪**Encephalitis** in **immunocompromised**, especially **AIDS**. Manifest by neurological signs from multiple **mass lesions**, usually in **basal ganglia**. Often relapses after treatment, can be **fatal**.
▪**Congenital Toxoplasmosis:** child spontaneously aborted; stillborn; born with encephalitis; or born mentally retarded.
●Life Cycle:
    Oocysts = shed in feces, get ingested
    Tachyzoites=invasive intracellular trophozoite.
    Tissue cysts = persist in tissues for life.
●Infection:
    ▪**Zoonotic** transmission occurs via ingestion of:
    Oocysts in food contaminated by **cat feces**, or
    Tissue cysts in under-cooked meats (lamb, pork).
    ▪**Vertical** transmission: **transplacentally** when mother gets **1° infection** during pregnancy.
●Diagnosis: (~34% AIDS patients have *Toxo*.)
    (But only ~6% have CNS Lymphoma)
▪**CT scan:** (can distinguish *Toxo* from Lymphoma)
    -Non-contrast: hypodense, multiple lesions.
        (Lymphoma is hyperdense, and single)
    -Contrast: ring-enhances, multiple lesions.
        (Lymphoma ring-enhances, but single)
▪**Congenital:** CT scan shows **focal calcifications**.
▪**Serology of newborn** will show high **IgM** titer.
●Treatment: **Pyrimethamine** plus **sulfadiazine**
●Prevention: Avoid cats. Cook food well.

Plasmodium spp:
    P. falciparum
    P. malariae
    P. ovale (rare)
    P. vivax
●Disease: **Malaria:**
●Symptoms:
    Cycle of Fever/chills: Every 48 hrs for *vivax,ovale*.
        Every 72 hrs for *malariae*.
        Irregularly for *falciparum*.
    "Black-Water Fever" hemoglobinuria occurs due to severe *falciparum* **hemolytic anemia**.
●Life Cycle:
▪Asexual cycle in Humans:
    1° tissue phase: mosquito "injects" **sporozoites** which go to liver and mature into **tissue schizonts**.
    Blood phase: liver tissue schizonts burst; release **merozoites** into blood to infect RBCs (and to become trophozoites). These then mature into **blood schizonts** which burst to release more merozoites which infect more RBCs, etc.
    Note: Bursting RBCs corresponds to the **cycle of fever**.
    2° tissue phase: *ovale* and *vivax* can remain **latent** in the liver as **hypnozoites** for months and then reactivate; this explains **relapses**.
▪Sexual cycle in Mosquitoes:
    Some **gametocytes** develop in RBCs; then get released when the RBCs burst; then get ingested by mosquitoes during a bite; then merge to form **zygotes**. The zygotes mature then divide into **sporozoites** which go to the mosquito **salivary glands**, to be injected.

Babesia spp
●Disease: **Malaria-like** symptoms.
●Infection: **Vector-borne** transmission via **Tick** bite.
    Northeast USA, California, Europe.
●Diagnosis: Peripheral smear shows trophozoites within RBC's.
    Occurring in **pairs** (which resemble P. falciparum), and **tetrads** ("maltese cross") within RBC's. Giemsa stain.
●Treatment: Quinine plus Clindamycin.

●Transmission:
    Vector-borne via **mosquito** bite.
    Vertical transplacental in utero.
    Iatrogenic due to blood transfusion.
NOTE: People with **Sickle cell gene** or **Thalassemia** are resistant to malaria.
●Diagnosis:
    ▪**Peripheral smear:** RBCs contain:
        falciparum: small ring form trophozoites.
        "Banana" shape gametocyte (rare).
        malariae: large, single, band trophozoite.
        "Daisy" shape schizont.
        Ovale: large, single ring trophozoite; in big oval shape RBC; Schuffner dots
        vivax: large, single ring trophozoite; in reticulocytes; Schuffner dots. Schizonts with many merozoites.
    ▪**Labs:** ↓hemoglobin; ↓hematocrit.
●Treatment: (problematic due to resistant strains)
▪**Chloroquine:** blood phase, and prophylaxis
▪**Primaquine:** tissue phase, and 2° hypnozoites.
▪Antifolates for chloroquine resistant strains.
▪Antibiotics for chloroquine-antifolate resistance.
▪**IV Quinine** for acute life-threatening attack.

FLUKES   Just The Essentials.

FLUKE FEATURES:
- **Adhesive suckers.**
- **Short, flat** body.
- **Blind gut.**

SCHISTOSOMIASIS:

Schistosoma haematobium
- Infection of the <u>**veins**</u> of the <u>**bladder**</u> and sometimes esophagus: tissue destruction by eggs.
- <u>Life cycle</u>: **Snails**→ Human (**urine**)→ **Snails.**
- <u>Infection</u> occurs due to *S. haematobium* **cercariae penetrating the skin** while swimming in fresh water. Found in **south-east Asia.**
- <u>Diagnosis</u>: **Eosinophilia;**
  Urine sample: <u>ovum with terminal spine</u>
- <u>Treatment</u>: **Praziquantel**

Schistosoma japonicum
- Infection of the <u>**veins**</u> of the <u>**liver**</u> and sometimes esophagus: tissue destruction by eggs.
- <u>Life cycle</u>: **Snails**→ Human (**urine**)→ **Snails.**
- <u>Infection</u> occurs due to *S. japonicum* **cercariae penetrating the skin** while swimming in fresh water; mostly found in **south-east Asia.**
- <u>Diagnosis</u>: **Eosinophilia;**
  Stool sample: characteristic **ovum**
- <u>Treatment</u>: **Praziquantel**

Schistosoma mansoni
- Infection of the <u>**veins**</u> of the <u>**liver**</u> and sometimes esophagus: tissue destruction by eggs.
- <u>Life cycle</u>: **Snails**→ Human (**urine**)→ **Snails.**
- <u>Infection</u> occurs due to *S. mansoni* **cercariae penetrating the skin** while swimming in fresh water. Found in **south-east Asia.**
- <u>Diagnosis</u>: **Eosinophilia;**
  Stool sample: <u>ovum with large lateral spine</u>
- <u>Treatment</u>: **Praziquantel**

Note: **"Swimmer's itch"** is caused by non-human-infecting *Schistosomas*.

LIVER FLUKE:
Clonorchis sinensis: **Oriental Liver Fluke**
- Infection of the **bile ducts** leads to cholangitis and sometimes **cholangiocarcinoma.**
- <u>Life cycle</u>:
  Snail→ Fish(**scales**)→ Human (**feces**)→ **Snail.**
- <u>Infection</u> occurs due to ingestion of **encysted larvae** present on raw or undercooked **fresh-water fish.** Found in **south-east Asia.**
- <u>Diagnosis</u>: **Eosinophilia;**
  Stool sample: characteristic **ovum with operculum.**
- <u>Treatment</u>: **Praziquantel**

LUNG FLUKE:
Paragonimus westermani
- Infection begins in small intestines then penetrates through diaphragm to lung parenchyma
- <u>Life cycle</u>: **Snail**→ **Crab**→ Human (**feces**)→ **Snail.**
- <u>Infection</u> occurs due to ingestion of **encysted larvae** present on raw or undercooked **crab.** Found in **south-east Asia.**
- <u>Diagnosis</u>: **Eosinophilia;**
  Stool sample: characteristic **ovum with operculum.**
- <u>Treatment</u>: **Praziquantel**

TAPE WORMS Just The Essentials.

TAPEWORM FEATURES:
- **Scolex** = attachment head: (suckers, hooks, sucking grooves).
- **Long, flat body.**
- **Proglottids** = multiple segments (older ones become gravid).
- **No gut**: nutrients are absorbed through tapeworm skin.

PORK TAPEWORM

Taenia solium LARVAL CYSTS→Worms
- Infection of **small intestines** begins when the larval cysts (cysticerci) attach with **hooks** into the mucosa. The worm matures in the lumen to attain 15' length.
- Symptoms: **anorexia** and diarrhea.
- Life cycle: **Pigs**→ Human (**feces**)→ **Pigs**.
- Infection occurs due to ingestion of *T. solium* **larval cysts** (cysticerci) present in raw or undercooked **pork**.
- Found in **Mexico, Ecuador, Asia**.
- Diagnosis: **Eosinophilia**;
  Stool sample: characteristic **gravid proglottids/eggs**
- Treatment: **Praziquantel** or **Niclosamide** kills the worm, but does not kill the eggs; therefore **Laxatives** may be used to remove the dead worm and eggs.

Cysticercosis

Taenia solium EGGS→Larval cysts
- **CNS cysticercosis** is a space-occupying lesion due to the presence of larval cysts (**cysticerci**) in the CNS.
- Symptoms: **seizures**, mass effects, and focal neurological deficits. Cysts may be found elsewhere in the patient's body.
- Life cycle: Human (**feces**)→ **Humans**.
- Horizontal transmission occurs by ingesting *T. solium* **eggs or proglottids** present in human feces, the eggs hatch into larvae which break through the intestinal wall and travel via the bloodstream to the brain and elsewhere.
- Found in **Mexico, Ecuador, Asia**.
- Diagnosis: **Eosinophilia**; CT scan shows focal calcification.
- Treatment: **antiepileptics** must be given for seizures; **Praziquantel** to kill the larval cysts; **Steroids** to control the inflammation that arises as the larvae die.

BEEF TAPEWORM

Taenia saginata LARVAL CYSTS→Worms
- Infection of **small intestines** begins when the larval cysts (cysticerci) attach with **suckers** onto the mucosa. The worm matures in the lumen to 30' length.
- Symptoms: **anorexia** and diarrhea.
- Life cycle: **Cattle**→ Human (**feces**)→ **Cattle**.
- Infection occurs due to ingestion of *T. solium* **larval cysts** (cysticerci) present in raw or undercooked **beef**.
- Found in **Central and South America, Africa**.
- Diagnosis: **Eosinophilia**;
  Stool sample: characteristic **gravid proglottids/eggs**
- Treatment: **Praziquantel** or **Niclosamide** kill the worm, but does not kill the eggs; therefore **laxatives** may be used to remove the dead worm and eggs.

FISH TAPEWORM

Diphyllobothrium latum LARVAE→Worms
- Infection of **small intestines** begins when the larval cysts (cysticerci) attach with **sucking groove** onto the mucosa.
- Symptoms: **Megaloblastic Anemia** (*D. latum* takes up vitamin **B12**), **anorexia** and diarrhea.
- Life cycle:
  Copepods→ Fish(**flesh**)→ Human (**feces**)→ **Copepods**
- Infection occurs due to ingestion of *D. latum* **larvae** present in raw or undercooked **fresh-water fish**.
- Found in **North America, Europe, Japan**.
- Diagnosis: **Eosinophilia**;
  Stool sample: characteristic **operculated eggs**
- Treatment: **Praziquantel** or **Niclosamide**.

HYDATID CYSTS

Echinococcus granulosus (Dog Tapeworm)
- **Unilocular hydatid cyst** infection of **liver, lungs, or brain**: a single, large, fluid-filled cyst **which contains thousands scoleces**.
- Symptoms: indicative of infected site, mass effect.
- Life cycle: **Sheep**→ Dog (**feces**)→ **Sheep**.

  Humans (**dead-end host**)
- Infection occurs by ingesting *E. granulosus* **eggs** present in **dog feces**, the eggs hatch, break through the intestinal wall, and travel via the bloodstream to the **liver** and elsewhere.
- Found **Worldwide wherever sheep live** among dogs.
- Diagnosis: **Eosinophilia**; serology, radiology.
- Treatment: **Surgery**; careful not to disrupt the cyst and spread the infectious contents.

Echinococcus multilocularis
- **Multilocular hydatid cyst** infection of **liver**: multiple fluid-filled cysts **which contain scoleces**.
- Symptoms: jaundice.
- Life cycle: **Rodents**→ Fox (**feces**)→ **Rodents**.

  Humans (**dead-end host**)
- Infection occurs by ingesting *E. granulosus* **eggs** present in **fox feces**, the eggs hatch, break through the intestinal wall, and travel via bloodstream to the **liver**.
- Found **Worldwide wherever foxes live**.
- Diagnosis: **Eosinophilia**; serology, radiology.
- Treatment: **Surgery**; careful not to disrupt the cyst and spread the infectious contents.

ROUND WORMS Just The Essentials.

ROUNDWORM FEATURES:
- **Round**, of varying lengths.
- **Non-segmented**.
- **Mouth, gut and anus.**

INTESTINAL NEMATODES:
[Humans as Intermediary Host]
[Penetrate skin]:

Ancylostoma duodenale **Hook worm** of Old-world
Necator americanus **Hook worm** of the Americas
- <u>Symptoms</u>: pneumonitis, intestinal upset, anemia.
- <u>Infection</u>: **larvae** in soil **penetrate bare feet**:
Travel via blood to lungs; then to trachea; then swallowed.
They attach to intestinal wall, mature, and suck blood.
- <u>Diagnosis</u>: **Eosinophilia**; stool sample: eggs.
- <u>Treatment</u>: **Mebendazole**

Strongyloides stercoralis **Thread worm**
- <u>Symptoms</u>: abdominal pain, peri-**anal pruritus**.
Can be **fatal**, especially in immunocompromised patients.
- <u>Infection</u>: **larvae** in soil **penetrate bare feet**:
Travel via blood to lungs; then to trachea; then swallowed.
They burrow into intestinal wall, mature, and lay eggs.
- <u>Autoinfection</u>: The eggs travel with feces, some turn into
larvae and infect colon: the larvae penetrate colon wall,
travel via blood to lungs, then to trachea, then swallowed,
then burrow into intestinal wall and may disseminate.
- <u>Skin infection</u>: **larvae** that arrive at anus may burrow
into peri-anal skin to cause itchy rash.
- <u>Diagnosis</u>: **Eosinophilia**; stool sample: larvae.
- <u>Treatment</u>: **Thiabendazole**

INTESTINAL NEMATODES:
[Humans as Intermediary Host]
[Ingested]:

Ascaris lumbricoides *Largest intestinal nematode.*
Most common cause of **helminth** infection worldwide.
- <u>Symptoms</u>: pneumonitis, anorexia, and sometimes
intestinal obstruction.
- <u>Infection</u>: **fecal-oral**: ingested **eggs** hatch into **larvae**:
the larvae penetrate intestinal wall, travel via blood to
lungs, then to trachea, then swallowed, then back to
intestinal lumen where they mature but **do not attach**.
- <u>Diagnosis</u>: **Eosinophilia**; stool sample: eggs.
- <u>Treatment</u>: **Mebendazole**, or **Pyrantel pamoate**.

Enterobius vermicularis **Pin worm**
Most common cause of **helminth** infection in the USA.
- <u>Symptoms</u>: peri-**anal pruritus**, sometimes bed-wetting.
- <u>Infection</u>: **oral route**: ingested **eggs** hatch into **larvae**,
then mature and reside in the **colon**. After mating, female
pinworms travel to the anus (usually at night) to lay eggs.
This accounts for the **itchy anus**, and for the presence of
infective eggs in the environment. Common in children.
- <u>Diagnosis</u>: **Eosinophilia**; stool sample: shows **no eggs**;
"**tape test**" is done to collect eggs from peri-anal skin.
- <u>Treatment</u>: **Mebendazole**, or **Pyrantel pamoate**.

Trichuris trichiura **Whip worm**
- <u>Infection</u>: ingest eggs, become larvae, travel to **cecum**.
- <u>Diagnosis</u>: No eosinophilia; stool sample: eggs.
- <u>Treatment</u>: **Mebendazole**

EXTRAINTESTINAL LARVAE:
[Humans as Dead-End host]
[Penetrates skin]:

Ancylostoma caninum (Dog Hookworm)
Cutaneous Larvae Migrans
- <u>Symptoms</u>: Dog Hookworm larvae
penetrate skin and "creep" around to
cause painful, itchy rash.
- <u>Treatment</u>: topical Thiabendazole.

EXTRAINTESTINAL LARVAE:
[Humans as Dead-End host]:
[Ingested]:

Toxocara canis (Dog Ascarid)
Visceral or
Ocular Larvae Migrans
- <u>Infection</u>: Dog Ascarid eggs: ingested,
become larvae, travel, die in various
organs: hepatomegaly, blindness.
- <u>Treatment</u>: No effective treatment.

Trichinella spiralis
Trichinosis
- <u>Symptoms</u>: fever, diarrhea, myositis,
periorbital edema.
- <u>Infection</u>: from ingesting **larval cysts**
in undercooked **pig** (pork) or **bear** flesh.
Larvae travel via blood to **encyst** in
striated muscles ("nurse cells"), first in
Ocular muscles. Myocarditis can be fatal.
Occurs worldwide, all climates.
- <u>Diagnosis</u>: Muscle biopsy;
Eosinophilia
- <u>Treatment</u>: No effective treatment.

TISSUE NEMATODES
[Vector-Borne Larvae]:

Dirofilaria immitis (Dog heart worm) **Lung lesion**
- <u>Symptoms</u>: lung nodule forms as worm dies.
- <u>Vector</u>: mosquito deposits larvae; worldwide
- <u>Treatment</u>: self-limited.

Loa loa **Eye worm**
- <u>Symptoms</u>: worm crawls across eyeball.
- <u>Vector</u>: **biting fly** deposit larvae; Africa.
- <u>Treatment</u>: **Diethylcarbamazine (DEC)**, Surgery.

Onchocerca volvulus **River Blindness**
- <u>Symptoms</u>: skin nodules, itchy "**leopard**" **rash**.
Blindness results due to worms that travel through
the skin to the eye to cause scarring of cornea.
- <u>Vector</u>: **black fly** deposits larvae; tropical.
- <u>Treatment</u>: **Ivermectin**.

Wuchereria bancrofti **Filariasis, Elephantiasis**
Brugia spp **Filariasis, Elephantiasis**
- <u>Symptoms</u>: **obstruction of lymphatic vessels**:
Filariasis indicates acute and recurrent symptoms; but
Elephantiasis indicates chronic obstruction and edema.
Microfilariae circulate in host blood at **night**; but
remain in liver and lungs during the day.
- <u>Vector</u>: **mosquito** deposits larvae; tropical.
- <u>Treatment</u>: **Diethylcarbamazine (DEC)**.

TISSUE NEMATODES [Non-Vector, Larvae]:
Dracunculus medinensis **Guinea worm**
- <u>Symptoms</u>: skin nodules; skin ulcers. Tropical.
- <u>Infection</u>: due to ingestion of infected **copepods**
(in drinking water); **larvae** get released from copepod;
larvae break through intestinal wall, and travel to skin.
- <u>Treatment</u>: pretreat with **Metronidazole**, then slowly
wind the worm onto a stick while pulling it out of skin.

Chapter 23

PARASITE CROSS REFERENCE

INTRACELLULAR	INFECT THROUGH SKIN	HUMAN DEAD-END HOST	SNAIL-RELATED	INHALATION ROUTE	VECTOR-BORNE
Leishmania donovani *Trypanosoma cruzi* *Cryptosporidium spp* *Isospora spp* *Toxoplasma gondii* *Plasmodium spp* *Babesia spp*	*Schistosoma spp* *Ancylostoma spp* *Necator americanus* *Strongyloides stercoralis*	*Echinococcus spp* *Ancylostoma caninum* *Toxocara canis* *Trichinella spiralis* *Dirofilaria immitis*	All Flukes	*Pneumocystis carinii*	*Leishmania spp* (sand fly) *Trypanosoma cruzi* (reduviid bug) *Trypanosoma spp* (Tsetse fly) *Plasmodium spp* (mosquito) *Babesia* (tick) *Dirofilaria immitis* (mosquito) *Loa loa* (fly) *Onchocerca volvulus* (black fly) *Wuchereria bancrofti* (mosquito) *Brugia spp* (mosquito)
	SWIMMING-RELATED		**SEAFOOD-RELATED**		
	Naegleria fowleri *Acanthamoeba spp* *Schistosoma spp*		*Clonorchis sinensis* (fish scales) *Paragonimus westermani* (crab) *Diphyllobothrium latum* (fish flesh)		
TEMPERATURE TROPISM					
Leishmania spp			**COPEPOD-RELATED**		
			Diphyllobothrium latum *Dracunculus medinensis*		
Modified ACID-FAST STAIN			**CAT-RELATED**		
Cryptosporidium spp *Isospora spp*			*Toxoplasma gondii*		
MEGALOBLASTIC ANEMIA			**DOG-RELATED**		
Diphyllobothrium latum			*Echinococcus granulosus* *Ancylostoma caninum* *Toxocara canis* *Dirofilaria immitis*		

NOTE: 1. These light microscope color plates represent typical specimens(not ideal specimens) as encountered in clinical practice.
2. All of the color plates on this page are magnified to equal high power (except as noted) to allow meaningful comparison of relative sizes.

Parasite Cross Reference **144**

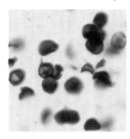

Pneumocystis carinii

Lung biopsy (GMS stain)

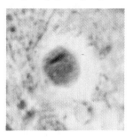

Entamoeba hystolytica

Cyst (with Chromatoid Bar Body).

Feces (Iron Hematoxylin stain)

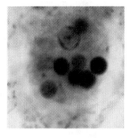

Entamoeba hystolytica

Trophozoite has ingested RBC's.

Feces (Iron Hematoxylin stain)

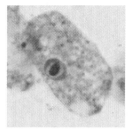

Acanthamoeba spp

Culture (Trichrome stain)

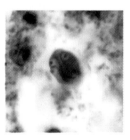

Giardia lamblia Cyst.

Feces (Iron Hematoxylin stain)

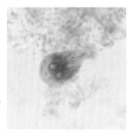

Giardia lamblia Trophozoite

Feces (Trochrome stain)

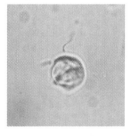

Trichomonas vaginalis

Vaginal wet mount

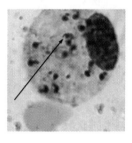

Leishmania donovani in Macrophage.

Bone marrow aspirate (Giemsa stain)

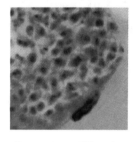

Trypanosoma cruzi Kinetoplasts

Heart biopsy (H&E stain)

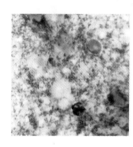

Cryptosporidium spp Oocytes

Feces (Modified Acid Fast stain)

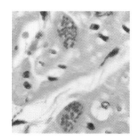

Toxoplasma gondii Cysts

Tissue biopsy (H&E stian)

Medium power view

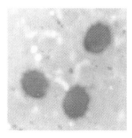

Toxoplasma gondii Trophozoites

Tissue biopsy (H&E stain)

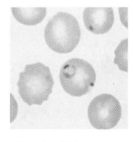

Plasmodium falcipoarum

Blood smear (Giemsa stain)

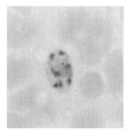

Plasmodium malariae

Bool smear (Giemsa stain)

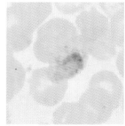

Plasmodium ovale

Blood smear (Giemsa stain)

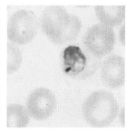

Plasmodium vivax

Blood smear (Giemsa stain)

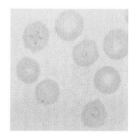

Babesia spp

Blood smear (Giemsa stain)

NOTE: 1. These light microscope color plates represent typical specimens(not ideal specimens) as encountered in clinical practice.
2. All of the color plates on this page are magnified to equal medium power to allow meaningful comparison of egg sizes.

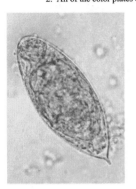

Shistosoma haematobium Egg

Feces

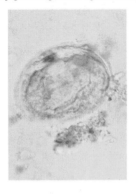

Shistosoma japonicum Egg

Feces

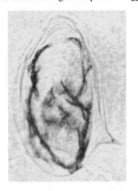

Shistosoma mansoni Egg

Feces

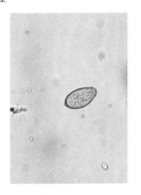

Clonorchis sinensis Egg

Feces

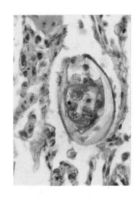

Paragonimus westermani Egg

Lung biopsy

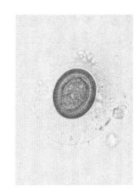

Taenia solium Egg

Feces

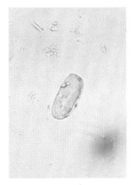

Ancylostoma duodenale Egg

Feces

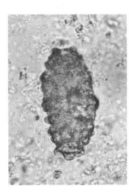

Ascaris lumbricoides

Infertile Egg

Feces

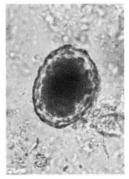

Ascaris lumbricoides

Fertile Egg

Feces

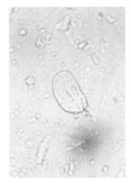

Enterobius vermicularis Egg

Feces

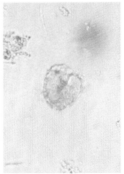

Enterobius vermicularis

Advanced Egg

Feces

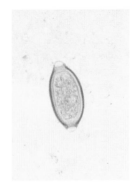

Trichuris trichiura Egg

Feces

Chapter 24

GENERAL CROSS REFERENCE (Part 1)

NORMAL FLORA [COMMENSALS]:
[Most common organisms only]
SKIN:
Staphylococcus spp
Streptococcus spp
Propionibacterium acnes
NOSE:
Staphylococcus aureus
MOUTH/THROAT:
Streptococcus Viridans Group
Non-gonococcal *Neisseria spp*
Non-Typeable *Haemophilus*
Candida
TEETH/GINGIVA:
Group D Streptococcus
Anaerobes:

Peptostreptococcus
Lactobacillus spp
Actinomyces israelii
Fusobacterium spp
Prevotella spp
STOMACH:
Some Gram POS Bacteria
INTESTINES:
Commensal Anaerobes especially
#1 *Bacteroides fragilis*
Enteric *E. coli*
Enterococcus spp
VAGINA:
Lactobacillus spp
Gardnerella vaginalis
Group B Streptococcus
E. coli
Candida

CAUSES OF MENINGITIS:
ASEPTIC (VIRAL)
#1: Picorna Enteroviruses
  Echo virus
  Coxsackie viruses
  Polio virus
#2: Mumps virus
#3: Herpes Simplex virus 2
#4: Lymphocytic
  choriomeningitis virus

BACTERIAL
#1: *Haemophilus influenzae*
  (especially children)
#2: *Neisseria meningitidis*
#3: *Streptococcus pneumoniae*
#4: *Listeria monocytogenes*

NEONATAL
#1: Group B Streptococcus
#2: *E. coli*
#3: *Listeria monocytogenes*

IMMUNOCOMPROMISED
#1: *Streptococcus pneumoniae*
#2: *Listeria monocytogenes*
ADULTS/ELDERLY
#1: *Streptococcus pneumoniae*
HEAD TRAUMA/SURGERY
#1: *Staphylococcus aureus*
CHRONIC MENINGITIS
Mycobacterium tuberculosis
Treponema pallidum
Borrelia burgorferi
Cryptococcus neoformans

MENINGITIS CSF FINDINGS:
VIRAL (ASEPTIC)
  Normal color
  Normal pressure
  ↑Proteins
  ↑Lymphocytes
  Slight ↓Glucose
(Herpes causes blood in CSF)
BACTERIAL
  Cloudy color
  ↑Pressure
  ↑Proteins
  ↑PMN leukocytes
  ↓↓↓Glucose
TUBERCULOUS
  Cloudy color
  ↑Pressure
  ↑Proteins
  ↑Lymphocytes
  ↓↓Glucose
CRYPTOCOCCUS
  Same CSF as tuberculosis
  India ink stain of CSF
SYPHILIS
  VRDL test of CSF
LYME DISEASE
  ↑Proteins
  ↑↑↑Lymphocytes
  Normal Glucose

NUCHAL SIGNS:
Nuchal rigidity (neck stiffness)
Brudzinski sign
Kernig sign

MENINGITIS TREATMENT:
VIRAL (ASEPTIC):
Symptomatic treatment only
NEONATAL BACTERIA:
Ampicillin plus Gentamicin

BACTERIA:
Haemophilus influenzae
  Cefotaxime,
  Ceftriaxone or
  Chloramphenicol
Neisseria meningitidis
  Penicillin G
Streptococcus pneumoniae
  Penicillin G

MENINGITIS PROPHYLAXIS:
1. **Ampicillin** Intrapartum IV
(Erythromycin in penicillin allergy)
if pregnant mother carries:
  Group B Streptococcus
2. **Rifampin** for contacts of:
  H. influenzae
  N. meningitidis

MENINGITIS PREVENTION:
1. **Mumps virus** vaccine
2. *H. influenzae type b* vaccine
  (very effective)
3. *N. meningitidis* vaccine
  (moderately effective)
4. *S. pneumoniae* vaccine
  (moderately effective)

GENERAL CROSS REFERENCE (Part 2)

PNEUMONIA:
COMMUNITY ACQUIRED:
Productive cough:
  Lobar pneumonia
  Bronchopneumonia
#1. *Streptococcus pneumoniae*
  (rusty sputum)
#2. *Haemophilus influenzae*
#3. *Staphylococcus aureus*

ATYPICAL Community acquired:
Dry, non-productive cough:
  Interstitial pneumonia:
#1. **Mycoplasma pneumoniae**
  (especially teenagers)
#2. **Chlamydia pneumoniae**
#3. *Coxiella burnetii*
#4. Viral:
  Influenza A and B
  Adenovirus 3, 4, 7
  (military)
  RSV (infants)
#5. *Legionella pneumophilia*
  (humidifiers, etc.)

IMMUNOCOMPROMISED:
[COPD, Diabetes, Alcoholism]:
Klebsiella pneumoniae
  (currant jelly sputum)
Pseudomonas aeruginosa

IN AIDS:
Pneumocystis carinii protozoa

IN CYSTIC FIBROSIS:
Pseudomonas aeruginosa

Post Viral URI Pneumonia:
Staphylococcus aureus

INFECTIVE ENDOCARDITIS:
SUB-ACUTE ENDOCARDITIS:
Chronic infection.
Fatal in 3-6 months.
Infects defective heart valves due to
  hematological spread,
Especially after dental work.
Left heart valves most common:
  mitral and/or aortic,
  grow valvular vegetations.
ORGANISMS:
#1. **Streptococcus Viridans Group**
#2. **Streptococcus Group D**
#3. *Enterococcus spp*
#4. *Staphylococcus epidermidis*
#5. *Salmonella spp*

ACUTE ENDOCARDITIS:
Fulminant infection.
Fatal in days to weeks.
Infects healthy heart valves or
  defective heart valves.
Left heart valves most common:
  mitral and/or aortic,
  grow valvular vegetations.
ORGANISMS:
#1. *Staphylococcus aureus*
#2. *Streptococcus pneumoniae*
#3. *Coxiella burnetii*

INFECTIVE ENDOCARDITIS
IN IV DRUG ABUSERS:
Right heart valves very common:
  especially tricuspid,
  grow valvular vegetations.
ORGANISMS:
#1. *Staphylococcus aureus*
#2. *Pseudomonas aeruginosa*
#3. *Candida spp*
#4. *Serratia marcescens*

"CULTURE NEGATIVE"
INFECTIVE ENDOCARDITIS:
Some important reasons why blood
cultures show no growth during
infective endocarditis:
#1. Prior treatment with antibiotics
#2. Organisms:
  Coxiella burnetii
  Brucella spp
  Chlamydia spp
  Fungi
"HACEK" organisms:
  Haemophilus spp
  Actinobacillus spp
  Cardiobacterium spp
  Eikenella spp
  Kingella spp

INFECTIVE MYOCARDITIS:
May be rapidly fatal within hours.
ORGANISMS:
#1. Coxsackie viruses
#2. Other Picornaviruses
#3. *Corynebacterium diphtheriae*
#4. *Trypanosoma cruzi* protozoa
  (Chagas disease)

ACUTE RHEUMATIC FEVER:
Pancarditis (affects all layers).
Auto-immune-mediated sequelae.
Follows pharyngitis infection by
Group A Streptococcus

RHEUMATIC HEART DISEASE
Cardiac valve deformities:
Chronic and progressive sequelae
(develops over years to decades)
from the auto-immune-mediated
post-pharyngeal infection by
Group A Streptococcus

CANCER ASSOCIATIONS:
Streptococcus Group D
  (Colon cancer)

Helicobacter pylori
  (Gastric carcinoma)

HPV-16, HPV-18
  (Cervical carcinoma)

HBV, HCV HDV
  (Hepatocellular carcinoma)

EBV
  (Burkett Lymphoma)
  (Nasopharyngeal carcinoma)

HTLV-1
  (T-cell Leukemia/Lymphoma)

HTLV-2
  (Hairy Cell Leukemia)

HIV
  (Kaposi sarcoma)
  (CNS Lymphoma)

Clonorchis sinensis fluke
  (Cholangiocarcinoma)

GENERAL CROSS REFERENCE (Part 3)

URINARY TRACT INFECTION:

(10^5 bacteria/ml urine)

Ascending route is most common
(via the urethra).

Common in women (short urethra)

CYSTITIS (bladder or lower UTI)
Most common UTI, no fever

PYELONEPHRITIS
(kidney or upper UTI)
Fever, back tenderness.

ORGANISMS:
#1. *Uropathogenic E. coli* (95%)
#2. *Proteus mirabilis*
others *Enterobacter cloacae*
Serratia marcescens
Klebsiella pneumoniae
Pseudomonas aeruginosa
Staph. saprophyticus
Enterococcus spp

HEMORRHAGIC CYSTITIS:
Adenovirus 11, 21

KIDNEY STONES:

(Nephrolithiasis, Urolithiasis)
(Struvite stones: triple phosphate =
ammonium magnesium phosphate);
(Renal calculi: Staghorn calculi).
#1. *Proteus mirabilis*
Others: *Proteus vulgaris*
Morganella morganii

SEPSIS:

#1. *Staphylococcus spp*
#2. *Streptococcus spp*

NOSOCOMIAL

BACTEREMIA:

#1. *Uropathogenic E. coli*
#2. *Klebsiella pneumoniae*
#3. *Pseudomonas aerginosa*
#4. *Enterobacter spp*
Other: *Yersinia enterocolitica*
(in multiple blood transfusions)
Providencia rettgeri
(in nursing home with catheter)

STDs:

[Sexually Transmitted Diseases]
[Most common organisms only]
#1. ***Chlamydia trachomatis***

BACTERIA:
Neisseria gonorrhoeae
(urethritis)
Treponema pallidum
(painless chancre)
(1°, 2°, 3° syphilis)
Chlamydia trachomatis
(urethritis)
(lymphogranuloma venereum)
Haemophilus ducreyi
(painful chancroid)
Calymmatobacterium granulomatis
(Donovanosis)
(granuloma inguinale)
Gardnerella vaginalis
("bacterial vaginosis")
(foul-odor discharge)
(wet mount: epithelial "clue cells")

VIRUSES:
HPV (condyloma acuminata)
HBV (hepatitis)
HSV-2 (herpes genitalis)
CMV (Mononucleosis)
EBV (Mononucleosis)
Molluscum contagiosum virus
(Poxvirus papule)
HTLV-1,-2 (malignancy)
HIV (AIDS)

FUNGI:
Candida albicans (yeast)

PARASITES:
Trichomonas vaginalis
(foul-odor discharge)

OTHER:
Phthirus pubis (Crab lice)
Sarcoptes scabiei (Scabies)

NEONATAL INFECTIONS:

#1. Group B Streptococcus
#2. *E. coli*

**ROUTES OF VERTICAL
TRANSMISSION:**
Transplacental in utero.
Ascending in utero.
Passage through vagina at birth.
Breast feeding.

"TORCH" ORGANISMS:
[Congenital neonatal infections]
[Transplacental vertical infection]
Toxoplasma gondii protozoa
OTHER:
Group B Streptococcus
(not transplacental)
Listeria monocytogenes
E. coli
(not transplacental)
Treponema pallidum
Parvo B19
HIV
Rubella virus
CMV
HSV (non-transplacental)

FROM BREAST FEEDING:
HBV
HTLV-1, HTLV-2
HIV

EYE INFECTIONS:
Neisseria gonorrhoeae
Chlamydia trachomatis

GENERAL CROSS REFERENCE (Part 4)

#1 CAUSATIVE ORGANISMS:

CELLULITIS:
#1. Group A Streptococcus
Other: *Pasteurella multocida*
(from cat/dog bite)

OTITIS MEDIA:
#1. *Streptococcus pneumoniae*
Others: Nontypeable *H. influenzae*
Moraxella catarrhalis

SINUSITIS:
#1. *Streptococcus pneumoniae*
#2. Nontypeable *H. influenzae*

EPIGLOTTITIS:
#1. *Haemophilus influenzae type b*
(must intubate immediately)

PERITONITIS:
#1. *Bacteroides fragilis*

OSTEOMYELITIS:
#1. *Staphylococcus aureus*
Note: *Salmonella spp* is common in patients with Sickle cell anemia.

INFECTIOUS ARTHRITIS:
#1. *Staphylococcus aureus*
Note: *Neisseria gonorrhoeae* causes monarticular infectious arthritis in sexually active young women.
Note: *Serratia marcescens* common from intra-articular injections.

PSEUDOAPPENDICITIS:
Salmonella spp
Campylobacter jejuni
Yersinia enterocolitica

REITER SYNDROME:
[Post-infectious autoimmune mediated arthritis; associated with HLA-B27 genotype]
Salmonella spp
Shigella spp
Campylobacter spp
Yersinia enterocolitica

REYE SYNDROME:
[Post-viral infection sequelae in children who use **aspirin** during viral infection]
#1. Influenza B
#2. Influenza A
#3. VZV

LIVE VACCINES (ATTENUATED):

BACTERIA:
Francisella tularensis
Mycobacterium (BCG)

VIRUSES:
Adenovirus 4, 7
VZV
Poxvirus (small pox)
Poliovirus (OPV)
Rubella (MMR)
Yellow Fever virus
Mumps (MMR)
Measles (MMR)

DEAD VACCINES (INACTIVATED):

BACTERIA:
Streptococcus pneumoniae
Neisseria meningitidis
Bordetella pertussis (DPT)
Haemophilus influenzae b (Hib)
Vibrio cholera
Bacillus anthracis
Yersinia pestis
Rickettsia prowazeckii

VIRUSES:
HBV
HAV
Poliovirus (IPV)
Japanese Encephalitis virus
Rabies (HDCV, RVA)
Influenza A and B

TOXOIDS:
Corynebacterium
diphtheriae (DPT)
Clostridium tetani (DPT)

VACCINES FOR ANIMALS:
Brucella spp
Leptospira interrogans
Toga encephalitis viruses
Eastern equine
Western equine
Venezuela

NOMENCLATURE CLARIFICATIONS:

"Coagulase Neg Staphylococcus" refers to **non** *S. aureus* Staphylococcus.

MRSA refers to "Methicillin-Resistant-*Staphylococus-aureu*s.

VRE refers to Vancomycin-Resistant-*Enterococcus*.

"Beta-hemolytic Streptococcus" refers to Group A Strep. (GAS) and Group B strep. (GBS).

Enterococcus is a distinct genus, not part of *Streptococcus*

Pneumococcus refers to Streptococcus pneumoniae.

Gonococcus refers to *Neisseria gonorrhoeae*

Meningococcus refers to *Neisseria meningitidis*

"Diphtheroids" refers to all non-*C. diphtheria* Corynebacteria.

Moraxella catarrhalis is new name for called *Branhamella catarrhalis*.

Bartonella is the new genus name for some bacteria formerly called *Rochalimaea*

"Non-typeable *H. influenzae*" refers to **non**-type b strains of "*H. flu*."

"AFB" refers to Acid-Fast Bacteria.

"Acid-fast" stain refers to Ziehl-Neelsen or Kinyoun stain.

"Modified Acid-fast" refers to similar stain without alcohol, but sometimes still called "Acid-fast."

"MAI" and "MAC" refer to Mycobacterium-Avium-Intracellulare Complex.

"Non-tuberculous" or "atypical" *Mycobacterium* refers to those strains which do not cause TB.

"Non A non B hepatitis" refers to HCV or HDV and sometimes HEV.

INDEX